The Complete Baby Name Guide

A Comprehensive Collection of Baby Names With Special Meanings, Origins, and Significance for Parents Seeking Unique, Timeless, and Culturally-Rich Names

Colton Blake

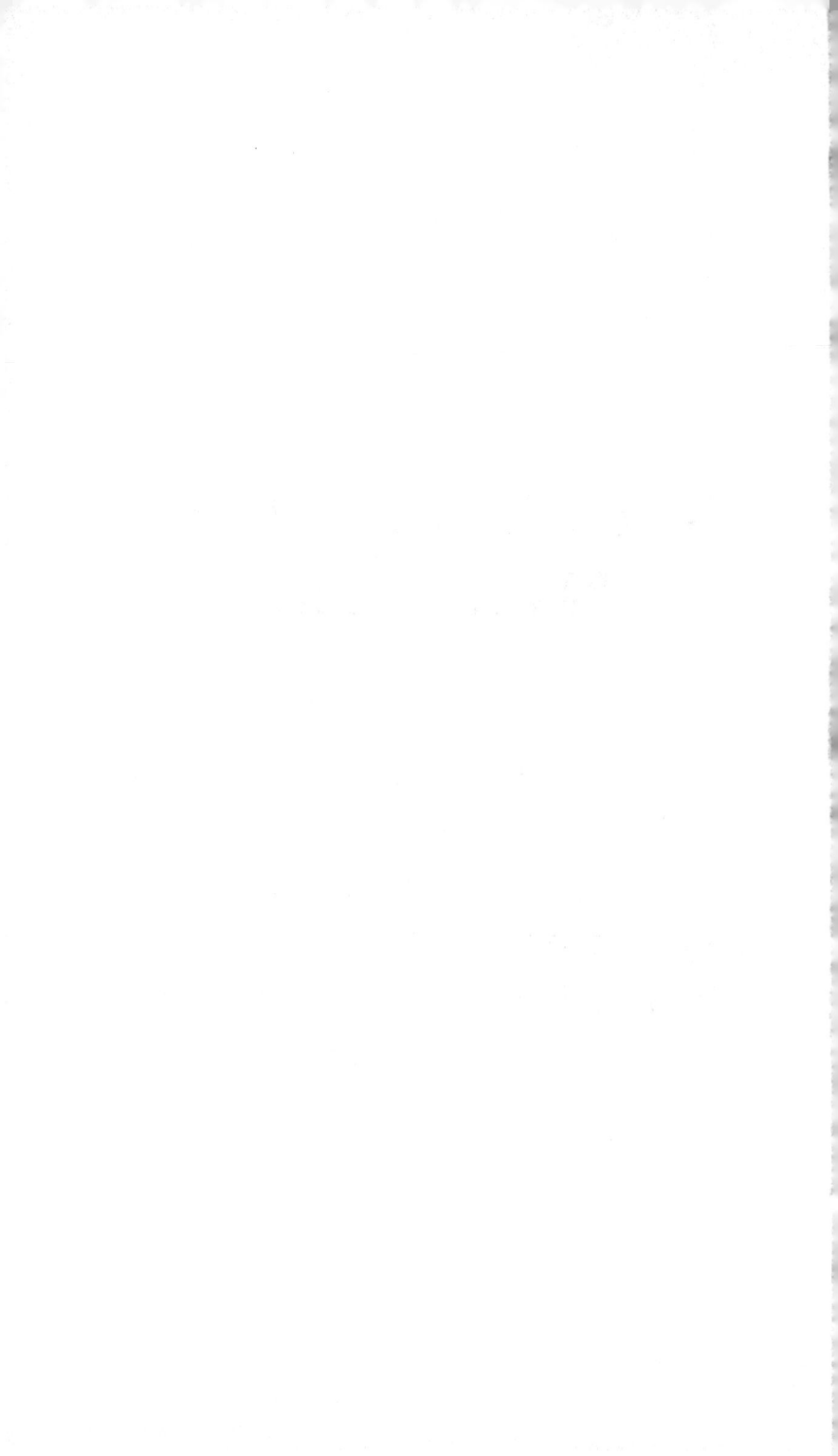

© Copyright 2024 - All rights reserved.

The content contained within this book may not be reproduced, duplicated or transmitted without direct written permission from the author or the publisher.

Under no circumstances will any blame or legal responsibility be held against the publisher, or author, for any damages, reparation, or monetary loss due to the information contained within this book, either directly or indirectly.

Legal Notice:

This book is copyright protected. It is only for personal use. You cannot amend, distribute, sell, use, quote or paraphrase any part, or the content within this book, without the consent of the author or publisher.

Disclaimer Notice:

Please note the information contained within this document is for educational and entertainment purposes only. All effort has been executed to present accurate, up to date, reliable, complete information. No warranties of any kind are declared or implied. Readers acknowledge that the author is not engaged in the rendering of legal, financial, medical or professional advice. The content within this book has been derived from various sources. Please consult a licensed professional before attempting any techniques outlined in this book.

By reading this document, the reader agrees that under no circumstances is the author responsible for any losses, direct or indirect, that are incurred as a result of the use of the information contained within this document, including, but not limited to, errors, omissions, or inaccuracies.

Table of Contents

INTRODUCTION 1
    How to Use This Guide 2

CHAPTER 1: THE ART OF CHOOSING THE PERFECT NAME 5
    THE MEANING BEHIND A NAME: A GATEWAY TO IDENTITY 6
        Names as Social Symbols 6
        Unforeseen Discoveries...7
        How Meaning Shapes Identity 7
        Names and Family Heritage..8
        Cultural and Historical Significance 9
    CHOOSING THE RIGHT MEANING AND IMPACT FOR YOUR CHILD'S NAME
   9
        Reflect on What Matters Most to You 10
        Explore Name Meanings and Qualities You Value...........10
        Honor Family Heritage..11
        Research Cultural and Historical Significance..................11
        Consider Social Perception...12
        Check for Practicality in Daily Use....................................13
        Timeless Appeal 13
        Test for Resonance With Your Identity.............................14
        Seek Input—But Trust Your Instincts................................14
        Using the Chapters Ahead 14

CHAPTER 2: TIMELESS AND CLASSIC BABY NAMES 17
    THE LONGEVITY OF CLASSIC NAMES 18
    CULTURAL AND HISTORICAL SIGNIFICANCE......................................24
    THE TIMELESS ELEGANCE OF SIMPLICITY..30

    Cross-Cultural Endurance 37
    Emotional and Familial Connections 41
    Wrapping Up...45

CHAPTER 3: UNIQUE AND RARE BABY NAMES......................47

    The Appeal of Unique Names 47
    Balancing Uniqueness With Practicality 53
    Rare Names With a Cultural and Global Perspective..............58
    Uncommon Names With Deep Meanings.................................64
    Wrapping Up...71

CHAPTER 4: NATURE-INSPIRED AND MYTHOLOGICAL NAMES 73

    The Appeal of Nature-Inspired Names 74
    Names Rooted in the Elements: Earth, Air, Fire, and Water 80
    Mythological Names With Powerful Meanings 84
    Wrapping Up...90

CHAPTER 5: MODERN AND GENDER-NEUTRAL NAMES.........91

    The Growing Popularity of Gender-Neutral Names 92
    Flexibility and Inclusivity of Gender-Neutral Names...............96
    Modern Names Reflecting Current Trends...........................101
    The Appeal of Simplicity and Versatility in Modern and Gender-Neutral Names 105
    Empowering Children With Names That Defy Stereotypes 108
    Wrapping Up...112

CHAPTER 6: SPIRITUAL, BIBLICAL, AND CULTURAL NAMES .113

    The Deep Meaning Behind Spiritual and Biblical Names.........114
    How Names Connect to Historical and Religious Figures 121
    Cultural Names That Honor Heritage and Tradition............127
    Wrapping Up...135

CHAPTER 7: NAMES INSPIRED BY PLACES AND TRAVEL.......137

PERSONAL AND EMOTIONAL CONNECTIONS TO PLACE NAMES 138
PLACE NAMES THAT EVOKE A SENSE OF ADVENTURE AND WANDERLUST 143
UNIQUE AND DISTINCTIVE NATURE OF PLACE-BASED NAMES........... 147
WRAPPING UP 151

CHAPTER 8: FINAL TIPS FOR CHOOSING THE RIGHT NAME..153

HOW THE NAME PAIRS WITH THE LAST NAME 153
THINK ABOUT NICKNAMES 155
TEST THE NAME IN SENTENCES 156
CONSIDER POPULARITY 157
SLEEP ON IT 158
IMAGINE HOW THEY WILL SHARE THE NAME'S STORY 159
INVOLVE SIBLINGS IN THE PROCESS 160
LET GO OF PERFECTION 161
WRAPPING UP 162

CHAPTER 9: BABY NAME LIST 165

BOY NAMES 165
GIRL NAMES 209
GENDER-NEUTRAL NAMES 260

REFERENCES 295

Introduction

Naming your child is one of the most meaningful steps in welcoming them into your life. Whether you have a few cherished ideas already or are starting fresh with an open mind, this guide is here to inspire and support you. Choosing a name is more than just a practical decision—it's a way to honor your values, celebrate your heritage, and give your child a name that feels uniquely theirs.

For years, I've been captivated by the profound impact of names. Each one carries a story—a blend of history, meaning, and personal significance. Through careful research and thoughtful insights, I've crafted this guide to help you approach the naming process with creativity, clarity, and confidence. My goal is to provide a resource that not only educates but also empowers you to find a name that resonates deeply with your family's journey.

This book is more than just a collection of names. It's a thoughtful companion designed to make the naming process as inspiring as it is rewarding. Inside you'll find:

- **A wide variety of name styles:** From timeless classics to modern, gender-neutral options as well as nature-inspired gems and culturally significant treasures, there's something for every parent's taste.

- **Rich meanings and origins:** Each name is accompanied by its backstory, offering deeper insight into its cultural and historical roots.

- **Practical advice:** Learn how to balance creativity with usability, test the sound and fit of a name, and ensure your choice feels just right in real-life contexts.

How to Use This Guide

The book is structured to guide you through every step of the naming process, beginning with helpful tips and reflections and ending with a robust A–Z name list for your final inspiration. Here's a brief overview:

- **Exploration and inspiration:** The first chapters dive into various naming styles and themes, from classic and elegant names to unique and creative options. These sections are designed to spark ideas and expand your perspective on what makes a name meaningful and enduring.

- **Practical guidance:** Throughout this guide, you'll find actionable tips to simplify decision-making. Whether it's considering the cultural significance of a name or testing how it pairs with your family name, these tools will help you make an informed choice.

- **A–Z baby name list:** The book concludes with an extensive alphabetical list of names, blending the traditional, the modern, and the unique into one easy-to-use resource. This section is perfect for browsing when you're ready to zero in on your favorites or are simply looking for fresh ideas.

Whether this is your first child or another beautiful addition to your family, this book is here to support you every step of the way. Remember, the goal isn't to find the "perfect" name—it's to find one that feels like the perfect fit for your child's story.

Let's begin this exciting journey together. Your child's story starts here.

Chapter 1:
The Art of Choosing the Perfect Name

You've just discovered you're about to welcome a new life into your world, and suddenly, choosing a name becomes a thrilling part of the journey. Family and friends may offer suggestions, and there's no shortage of names on lists and websites. But how do you choose one that isn't just popular or trendy, but truly meaningful—something that holds significance and feels right for your family and future child?

A name is a gift, one that can carry cultural significance, honor family history, or reflect values and aspirations for the future. In this chapter, we'll explore the factors that contribute to a meaningful name, from its origins and cultural or historical roots to finding the balance between uniqueness and practicality. By thoughtfully considering these elements, you can choose a name that embodies your family's identity and the qualities you wish to nurture in your child.

The Meaning Behind a Name: A Gateway to Identity

When it comes to naming, many people start with the basics—how it sounds, whether it's easy to pronounce, or if it's popular. But going deeper, a name often carries a purpose or story that can shape a child's identity and connect them to their heritage.

Names as Social Symbols

Names often signify social, cultural, or educational backgrounds. Sociologists observe that names can act as markers within society, subtly influencing how individuals are perceived. For example, in France during the 1980s, names like Jennifer and Dylan gained popularity due to TV characters but were rarely chosen by families with higher educational backgrounds. These choices reflected broader social trends, demonstrating how names can sometimes hint at socioeconomic or educational status (Vincentelli, 2007).

While such patterns vary across cultures, they reveal the layered meanings names can carry. Beyond personal preferences, names have the power to influence first impressions, often before an individual even speaks.

Unforeseen Discoveries

Sometimes, parents may choose a name for its appeal, only to later uncover its deeper meaning. For instance, naming a child Liam for its simplicity might lead to the joyful discovery that it means "strong-willed warrior" in Irish. Such revelations can add emotional weight to the choice, enhancing its significance.

However, not all discoveries are positive. A name like Mallory, chosen for its pleasant sound, might later reveal its Old French meaning—"unfortunate"—causing some parents to question their decision (Moss, 2024). Similarly, historical or cultural associations can transform perceptions of a name over time. In Germany, the once-common name Adolf became heavily stigmatized post-World War II, leading to its near disappearance. These examples highlight the importance of understanding a name's history to ensure it aligns with parental intentions and values.

How Meaning Shapes Identity

A name with a positive meaning can play a crucial role in shaping a child's identity and self-esteem. Psychologists suggest that names influence how individuals perceive themselves and how they are treated by others, impacting their confidence and social interactions (McAndrew, 2020).

For example, in Japanese tradition, names often reflect virtues or elements of nature, such as Hana ("flower") for beauty or Hinata ("sunflower") for positivity (Thompson, 2024). Similarly, in Hindu culture, names like Aarav ("peace") or Lakshmi ("prosperity") embody traits parents hope their children will develop (Sharmaa, 2023). Across cultures, names are chosen to inspire qualities like kindness, resilience, or intelligence, offering children a sense of pride and connection.

Names and Family Heritage

A name can connect a child to their family's history and traditions, serving as a bridge between generations. For immigrant families, names often reflect cultural roots, helping children maintain ties to their heritage even when growing up far from their ancestral homeland.

For example, Irish-American families might choose names like Sean or Bridget to honor their origins, while Jewish families might use a Hebrew name like Ari alongside a secular name to balance cultural pride with daily practicality (McAndrew, 2020). These choices help foster a sense of belonging and pride in one's background.

Naming traditions, such as namesaking, further emphasize family connections. Naming a child after a relative or ancestor strengthens familial bonds and ensures the continuation of a legacy. Modern parents often balance these traditions with contemporary trends, blending ancestral names with unique touches to create a harmonious blend of history and individuality.

Cultural and Historical Significance

Throughout history, names have reflected societal values, beliefs, and aspirations. Selecting a name with cultural or historical significance allows parents to connect their child to a broader narrative.

Consider names inspired by historical figures or literary giants, such as Alexander (strength and leadership) or Dante (intellectual and artistic depth). These choices link children to stories of resilience, creativity, and ambition, fostering a sense of pride in their heritage.

Similarly, names from indigenous or regional traditions often carry symbolic meanings tied to nature, spirituality, or values like courage and love. Mythological or biblical names, such as Athena ("wisdom") or David ("faith"), offer timeless qualities that transcend cultural boundaries, grounding children in a sense of purpose and connection.

Choosing the Right Meaning and Impact for Your Child's Name

Now that we've explored how names can carry meaning, connect to family heritage, or embody cultural significance, you may feel inspired to consider the impact your child's name could have. Each aspect—symbolism in society, shaping identity, linking to family roots, and historical or cultural depth—offers something special. The following guide will help you make intentional choices and craft a name that reflects your values and hopes.

Reflect on What Matters Most to You

Start by considering what feels most important in a name. Does it need to reflect your cultural background or family traditions? Or are you drawn to names with positive meanings, such as those symbolizing kindness or resilience?

For some, family heritage is a priority. Explore existing naming traditions—like passing names down through generations or blending cultural names with secular ones. Others may find inspiration in historical figures, myths, or legends that align with their values or aspirations for their child.

Take time to reflect on these aspects. Doing so ensures your choice resonates with your family's identity and the future you envision for your child.

Explore Name Meanings and Qualities You Value

Every name holds meaning, whether subtle or profound. Look for names that embody qualities you cherish, like courage, intelligence, or harmony. Many cultures have names deeply tied to specific traits. For example, many African names emphasize strength and resilience, while certain Asian names may focus on harmony and balance. European names frequently derive from historical or mythological roots, symbolizing bravery or wisdom.

List values that are meaningful to you, then research names that represent those traits. Selecting a name that reflects these qualities can feel rewarding, as it nurtures the idea that they'll become part of your child's story.

Honor Family Heritage

A name can beautifully honor family heritage, creating a bridge to the past and grounding your child in a sense of continuity. For immigrant families, cultural names provide a lasting connection to their roots, even in new environments.

One approach is to blend traditional and modern names. For instance, pairing a classic family name as a middle name with a contemporary first name can celebrate history while offering a fresh touch. Alternatively, you might adapt a beloved ancestor's name to suit modern tastes.

These choices not only honor heritage but also create a meaningful connection for your child, helping them feel pride in their family's story.

Research Cultural and Historical Significance

Names from different cultures or historical eras carry depth and symbolism. Choosing a name tied to a culture or a historical figure you admire can provide an enduring connection for your child.

For example, mythological names like Athena ("wisdom") or Apollo ("creativity") carry symbolic resonance, while literary names like Dante or Eleanor reflect intellectual heritage. Similarly, biblical names like Miriam or David embody values tied to faith and virtue.

Researching names from various traditions can be an enjoyable journey, offering insights into stories, beliefs, and values that might inspire the life you envision for your child.

Consider Social Perception

Names influence how others perceive us, often before we even speak. Studies show that children with highly unusual names may face social challenges, as peers or teachers might struggle with pronunciation or form assumptions about their background (McAndrew, 2020).

While unique names can stand out, they may create unintended barriers. Striking a balance is key. For instance, names like Kai or Lia are distinctive yet simple to pronounce, offering uniqueness without complexity. You can choose a name that both resonates with you and supports your child's interactions throughout life by understanding potential social implications.

Check for Practicality in Daily Use

A name should be easy to live with. Even the most meaningful name may cause frustration if frequently mispronounced or difficult to spell.

Consider whether the name is straightforward to pronounce and remember. Test how it sounds when said aloud and how it pairs with a middle or last name. For instance, while a name like Saoirse (Irish for "freedom") has a beautiful meaning, its pronunciation (*Sur-sha*) might be unfamiliar in many settings.

It's also worth thinking about potential nicknames or variations. Most names evolve in casual use, so ensuring you're comfortable with these variations can help you feel confident in your choice.

Timeless Appeal

Names carry associations that may change over time. A name that feels trendy today could seem dated decades later, while classics often endure across generations.

For example, names like Elizabeth or Daniel are timeless, reflecting qualities that remain relevant regardless of era. On the other hand, names tied to specific periods—such as Barbara or Gary, popular in past decades—may feel less current to new generations.

Considering how a name might age ensures it remains a positive source of pride for your child as they grow.

Test for Resonance With Your Identity

Choosing a name that resonates with you as a parent is a deeply meaningful experience. This name reflects not only your dreams for your child but also your own values and cultural identity.

Ask yourself if the name brings you joy and pride. If it does, it's likely to bring the same feeling to your child. A name with personal significance, whether through family ties, shared values, or its sound, strengthens the connection between you and your child.

Seek Input—But Trust Your Instincts

Feedback from family or friends can enrich your naming journey, particularly when exploring cultural or family traditions. However, remember that the final decision should feel right to you.

Input on practical aspects, such as pronunciation or flow, can be helpful. Family members may also provide insights into cultural meanings or stories tied to certain names. Ultimately, these discussions can deepen your understanding, but your instincts should guide the final choice.

Using the Chapters Ahead

As you move into the upcoming chapters, you'll find a rich collection of names spanning timeless classics, nature-inspired choices, modern favorites, and culturally significant options. Each chapter offers an opportunity to explore names that might align with the hopes, values, or unique qualities you envision for your child.

Consider the story of Dana and Will, a couple who began their naming journey with a long list of nature-inspired names. They imagined a peaceful, nature-rooted name for their child, something like Willow or River. But as they worked through their list and discussed what felt right, they found themselves returning to a timeless classic, Amelia. To their surprise, Amelia had all the qualities they hoped for—a sense of strength, beauty, and elegance they wanted to convey. Naming, as they learned, is as much about finding the right feeling as it is about following any particular category.

As you go through each section, here are a few pointers to help you enjoy the process and get the most out of this guide:

- **Let curiosity lead the way:** Skim through names that catch your interest, letting your instincts guide you. A name might resonate simply because it feels right, or it may have a meaning or sound that aligns with the dreams you hold for your child.

- **Combine elements for a unique choice:** Don't be afraid to blend ideas from different chapters. Like Dana and Will, you may start with one vision and find that a blend of classic and modern or nature-inspired and timeless feels just right. Pairing influences helps you create a name that is truly one of a kind.

- **Focus on the values and qualities you want to embrace:** Each chapter includes names with meanings that reflect different qualities—strength, peace, curiosity, and kindness, among others. Note the names that align with the traits you hope your child will carry and see which combinations feel meaningful to you.

- **Take your time and enjoy the journey:** Naming is a process to savor. Each chapter invites you to explore a variety of names, each with cultural depth, modern appeal, or natural beauty. A thoughtfully chosen name offers your child more than just a label; it tells a story, shares a connection, and reflects values close to your heart.

Remember, whatever name you choose, it will be a beautiful beginning to your child's unique path. This name will be a cherished part of their identity and a lasting gift from you. So, take your time, trust your instincts, and enjoy the adventure.

Chapter 2:
Timeless and Classic Baby Names

As you search for the perfect name, there's something undeniably appealing about the classics. These are the names that have been spoken with pride, love, and admiration for generations. They carry a certain weight and a sense of tradition that feels both familiar and comforting. They also offer a connection to the past, bridging generations in a way that feels deeply rooted yet still fresh.

If you're looking for a name with elegance, simplicity, and lasting appeal, timeless classics have a lot to offer. In this chapter, we'll explore the many dimensions of classic names, from their deep cultural significance to the beauty of their simplicity.

All name origins and details provided here and in other chapters are sourced from Parents.com and TheBump.com, both of which thoroughly fact-check their information. We have also verified these sources to ensure accuracy. You'll see why these names have stood the test of time and how they bring a touch of tradition, heritage, and dignity to the people who carry them.

The Longevity of Classic Names

Classic names thrive where trends fade. They carry a sense of dependability, balancing familiarity with versatility. Whether chosen for their association with royalty, cultural icons, or enduring values, these names remain timeless because they feel equally fitting for a child or an adult.

Names like Elizabeth, James, and William are steeped in history. They've been borne by influential figures across centuries, from royalty to reformers, embodying qualities like strength, kindness, and resilience. Their adaptability across cultures and languages further solidifies their universal appeal.

For example:

- **Aaron:** A Hebrew name meaning "high mountain" or "exalted," Aaron reflects leadership and strength, famously borne by the brother of Moses in biblical tradition.

- **Alan:** Of Celtic origin, meaning "handsome" or "cheerful," Alan conveys approachability and charm. Its variants, such as Allan and Alun, make it a flexible and enduring choice.

- **Anthony:** Derived from Roman *Antonius* ("priceless one"), Anthony is enriched by its connection to Saint Anthony of Padua. Nicknames like Tony and Anton lend it a contemporary edge.

- **Charles:** Meaning "free man," Charles is associated with influential figures like Charlemagne and Charles Darwin. Nicknames such as Charlie and Chuck offer a modern touch.

- **Charlotte:** Of French and German origin, Charlotte means "free man," derived from its masculine root. Associated with royalty, including Queen Charlotte, it symbolizes elegance and grace. Its versatility, with nicknames like Charlie and Lottie, adds to its enduring charm.

- **Dominic:** Dominic, meaning "of the Lord," has roots in Latin and ties to Saint Dominic. Its strong yet versatile nature makes it a favorite across cultures and languages. Nicknames like Dom and Nico add to its enduring charm.

- **Elizabeth:** Originating from Hebrew *Elisheva* ("God is my oath"), this name has enduring biblical and royal ties, most famously through Queen Elizabeth I and II. Variants like Isabel and Eliza, alongside nicknames such as Liz and Beth, highlight its versatility and timeless appeal.

- **Emily:** Derived from Latin *Aemilia* ("rival" or "eager"), Emily reflects ambition and charm. Its diminutives, such as Em and Milly, make it both versatile and endearing.

- **Emma:** A Germanic name meaning "whole" or "universal," Emma became popular through Queen Emma of Normandy and Jane Austen's

Emma. Its simplicity and elegance have cemented its global popularity.

- **Frederick:** Of Germanic origin, meaning "peaceful ruler," Frederick is tied to leaders like Frederick the Great. Nicknames like Fred and Freddie balance formality with friendliness.

- **George:** Derived from the Greek *Georgios* ("farmer"), George is tied to Saint George and English royalty. International variations, including Jorge and Giorgio, underscore its global appeal and historical significance.

- **Gregory:** From the Greek *Gregorios*, meaning "watchful" or "alert," Gregory honors Saint Gregory the Great. Variants like Gregor and the nickname Greg strike a balance between formality and friendliness.

- **Henry:** Meaning "house ruler," Henry has been a royal favorite across Europe. Nicknames like Harry and Hank add a friendly vibe, while variations like Henri and Enrique show its adaptability.

- **Irene:** A Greek name meaning "peace," Irene is tied to the goddess Eirene and exudes tranquility. Variants like Irina and Irena give it a multicultural appeal across generations.

- **James:** From Hebrew *Ya'aqov* ("supplanter"), this classic name is rooted in biblical tradition and royal history. Its approachable nicknames,

Jim and Jamie, add to its universal charm and longevity.

- **Jessica:** Of Hebrew origin, meaning "rich" or "God beholds," Jessica gained fame through Shakespeare's *The Merchant of Venice*. Its nicknames, Jess and Jessie, enhance its charm and versatility.

- **Jillian:** A variant of the Latin name Juliana, Jillian means "youthful" or "dedicated to Jove." Its enduring popularity lies in its friendly charm and versatile nicknames like Jill. Jillian balances vintage appeal with modern adaptability.

- **Laura:** From Latin *laurus*, meaning "laurel," Laura signifies victory and honor and is famously tied to Petrarch's muse. Its timeless beauty makes it a consistent favorite.

- **Lucy:** Of Latin origin, meaning "light," Lucy is linked to radiance and vitality. Popularized by the Normans, variations like Lucia and Lucey add cultural richness to this beloved name.

- **Mason:** Once a British occupational surname for stoneworkers, Mason exudes strength and reliability. Widely used, Mason bridges the gap between classic and contemporary naming trends.

- **Melanie:** Derived from Greek *melas* ("dark"), Melanie offers a soft, timeless beauty. Its popularity rose through Saint Melanie, reflecting its historical significance. With an elegant simplicity, Melanie continues to captivate in modern times.

- **Melissa:** Meaning "honeybee," Melissa originates from Greek mythology, symbolizing sweetness. Its mythological ties to nurturing figures like the nymph Melissa enrich its depth. A melodious and widely used name, it retains its charm across generations.

- **Michelle:** A French feminine form of Michael, Michelle means "who is like God?" Its elegance and association with strong, iconic figures enhance its appeal. This classic name blends sophistication with a modern, approachable charm.

- **Nicole:** A feminine form of Nicholas, meaning "victory of the people," Nicole has a modern, elegant feel. Nicknames like Nikki and Cole add a contemporary touch to this classic name.

- **Olivia:** With Latin roots tied to the olive tree, Olivia symbolizes peace and beauty. Popularized through Shakespeare's *Twelfth Night*, it continues to captivate with its natural elegance.

- **Richard:** Of Germanic origin, meaning "brave ruler" or "powerful leader," Richard reflects leadership through figures like Richard the Lionheart. Familiar nicknames, including Rich and Rick, add to its lasting charm.

- **Robert:** A Germanic name meaning "bright fame," Robert has been borne by kings and historical figures. Nicknames like Rob, Robbie, and Bob give it an approachable and enduring charm.

- **Stephen:** Of Greek origin, meaning "crown" or "garland," Stephen is tied to Saint Stephen, the first Christian martyr. Variants like Steven and Stefan, along with the nickname Steve, ensure its timeless appeal.

- **Thomas:** From Aramaic *Ta'oma* ("twin"), Thomas is tied to Saint Thomas the Apostle and historical figures like Thomas Jefferson. Its nicknames Tom and Tommy bring warmth and approachability.

- **Victor:** Of Latin origin, meaning "conqueror" or "victorious," Victor is a name of strength and triumph. Its historical and cultural significance adds to its timeless charm. Victor's bold and confident sound ensures its enduring popularity.

- **Victoria:** From Latin *victoria* ("victory"), this regal name honors Queen Victoria and symbolizes strength and triumph. Nicknames like Vicky and Tori offer warmth and balance to its dignified heritage.

- **William:** With Germanic origins, meaning "resolute protector," William has historical significance through figures like William the Conqueror. Modern nicknames like Will, Liam, and Billy make it adaptable across cultures and eras.

These names endure because they adapt to changing times while maintaining their intrinsic charm. Their strength lies in their ability to resonate across generations, making them reliable companions through all stages of life.

Cultural and Historical Significance

Classic names often carry a rich cultural and historical narrative. They are linked to influential figures—leaders, intellectuals, and artists—who shaped history and inspired values like wisdom, courage, and resilience. Choosing a name like Alexander or Eleanor connects your child to these stories, instilling a sense of heritage and purpose.

Examples include:

- **Adrian:** Derived from the Latin *Hadrianus*, meaning "from Hadria," Adrian has historic ties to Roman emperors and saints. It symbolizes strength and sophistication, with variants like Adrien (French) and nicknames like Ade adding versatility.

- **Alexander:** Greek for "defender of men," this name symbolizes courage and leadership and is famously associated with Alexander the Great. Variants like Alejandro, Alessandro, and

Alexandre as well as nicknames such as Alex, Lex, and Xander enhance its adaptability.

- **Alexandra:** Alexandra, or Alessandra, is a feminine form of Alexander, which means "defender of men." It exudes grace. With roots in Greek mythology and royal history, it is elegant and versatile, offering nicknames like Alex, Lexi, and Sandra.

- **Andrew:** Greek for "manly" or "courageous," Andrew is tied to strength and faith, with biblical roots as Jesus's first Apostle. Variations like Andre make it a globally versatile and honorable choice.

- **Arnold:** Derived from Old German, Arnold means "eagle power." It reflects strength and resilience and is historically tied to leaders and warriors. Arnold's vintage charm is complemented by its strong, commanding sound.

- **Arthur:** Likely derived from Celtic *artos* ("bear") or Latin *artorius* ("noble one"), Arthur evokes nobility and bravery as inspired by the legendary King Arthur. Nicknames like Art and Artie modernize its charm, while variations like Arturo add a cultural twist.

- **Beatrice:** Latin for "voyager" or "blessed," Beatrice symbolizes joy and inspiration, famously represented in Dante's *Divine Comedy*. Its timeless sophistication makes it ideal for a child with a bright, adventurous spirit.

- **Bruce:** Of Scottish origin, Bruce means "from the brushwood thicket." It evokes strength and nobility and is famously tied to Robert the Bruce, King of Scotland. Bruce's timeless and rugged appeal makes it a bold, classic choice.

- **Catherine:** Greek for "pure," Catherine has been borne by queens, saints, and other influential figures, symbolizing virtue and resilience. Variations like Katherine and nicknames like Kate and Cathy make it timelessly versatile.

- **Cecilia:** From the Latin *Caecilius*, meaning "blind," Cecilia carries a timeless charm. Associated with Saint Cecilia, the patron saint of music, it symbolizes creativity and devotion. Nicknames like Cece and Cilla add warmth to this classic name.

- **Clarence:** Derived from the Latin *Clarus*, meaning "bright" or "clear," Clarence gained popularity through its royal and noble associations. It is a distinguished name with a vintage charm, offering nicknames like Clare and Clarry.

- **Diana:** Latin for "divine," Diana reflects strength and grace, rooted in Roman mythology as the goddess of the hunt. Princess Diana's legacy adds modern elegance and compassion to this timeless choice.

- **Eleanor:** Meaning "shining light," Eleanor is tied to powerful figures like Eleanor of

Aquitaine and Eleanor Roosevelt. Nicknames Ellie and Nora, along with variants like Elinor, offer modern flair while retaining its historical gravitas.

- **Fiona:** Of Gaelic origin, Fiona means "fair" or "white." It gained prominence through Scottish poetry and literature. Elegant and refined, Fiona carries a sense of timeless beauty.

- **Genevieve:** Meaning "woman", "family," or "white fay," Genevieve has French, Germanic, and Welsh roots. It is tied to Saint Genevieve, the patron saint of Paris, symbolizing strength. The name's historical and cultural depth enhances its enduring appeal.

- **Helen:** Meaning "torch" or "light" in Greek, Helen is epitomized by Helen of Troy's legendary beauty. Variations like Elena and Helena add international elegance, symbolizing grace and allure.

- **Joshua:** A Hebrew name meaning "God is salvation," Joshua is tied to the biblical figure who led the Israelites into the Promised Land. It symbolizes faith, strength, and leadership. Nicknames like Josh make it approachable, ensuring its timeless and enduring appeal.

- **Julian:** Of Latin origin, Julian means "youthful" or "downy-bearded." Associated with historical and religious figures, it offers cultural versatility through variations like Julien (French) and

Giuliano (Italian). Nicknames like Jules add charm, making it a sophisticated choice.

- **Juliette:** A French diminutive of Julia, this name means "youthful" or "soft-haired." Romanticized by Shakespeare's *Romeo and Juliet*, it embodies elegance. Its lyrical sound and cultural resonance ensure it remains a classic favorite.

- **Lawrence:** Derived from the Latin *Laurentius*, meaning "from Laurentum," Lawrence is tied to victory through the laurel tree. Known for its strength and refinement, it has variations like Laurence and Lorenzo.

- **Louis:** From the Germanic *Ludwig* ("renowned warrior"), Louis is a name of French royalty. Nicknames like Lou and Louie, along with feminine forms like Louise and Lulu, add warmth to its noble roots.

- **Lucia:** Derived from the Latin *lux,* meaning "light," Lucia has deep European roots. Celebrated in Italian and Spanish traditions, it symbolizes radiance and hope. Its timeless charm and adaptability make it a beloved name across generations.

- **Miles:** Latin for "soldier," Miles represents strength and kindness. Popularized by figures like jazz legend Miles Davis, it blends historical depth with modern heroism, offering an approachable yet classic feel.

- **Oscar:** Of Irish origin, meaning "friend of deer" or "warrior," Oscar is tied to Irish mythology through the hero Oisín's son. It also has Scandinavian roots, symbolizing strength and nobility. Popularized by literary icons like Oscar Wilde, the name carries both charm and timeless appeal.

- **Patrick:** From the Latin *Patricius*, meaning "nobleman," Patrick is associated with Saint Patrick, the patron saint of Ireland. It symbolizes faith, heritage, and resilience. Nicknames like Pat, Paddy, and Rick offer versatility, making it a beloved name across cultures.

- **Rebecca:** A Hebrew name meaning "to bind" or "captivating," Rebecca is a biblical classic tied to strength and beauty. Nicknames like Becca and Becky lend a playful, approachable quality, making it a timeless and beloved choice.

- **Sophia:** Greek for "wisdom," Sophia embodies intelligence and beauty. Variations like Sophie maintain its elegance, while its philosophical and royal connections ensure universal admiration.

- **Susanna:** From the Hebrew *Shoshannah*, meaning "lily," Susanna symbolizes purity and grace. Variations like Suzanne (French) and Susan offer cultural versatility, while nicknames like Susie and Anna add charm and warmth.

- **Theodore:** Greek for "gift of God," Theodore gained prominence through figures like President Theodore Roosevelt. Nicknames like Theo and Teddy balance its dignity with warmth, making it a name of enduring strength and charm.

- **Veronica:** Of Latin origin, meaning "true image," Veronica has biblical ties through Saint Veronica, known for her compassion. It exudes elegance and resilience, with nicknames like Ronnie and Vera providing a contemporary flair.

- **Vincent:** From the Latin *Vincentius*, meaning "conquering" or "prevailing," Vincent exudes elegance and strength. It is tied to Saint Vincent and artistic figures like Vincent van Gogh. Vincent's refined tone and versatility make it a classic, enduring name.

Classic names with historical depth serve as more than a nod to tradition—they offer a narrative that encourages children to connect with values of strength, honor, and perseverance.

The Timeless Elegance of Simplicity

One reason classic names captivate is their simplicity. Names like Jane, Mark, and Rose are easy to say, spell, and remember. Their understated elegance transcends trends, offering a timeless quality that grows beautifully with the person who carries them.

Simple names convey reliability and strength. They aren't tied to fleeting fashions, making them feel appropriate in any era or setting.

For instance:

- **Abigail:** Hebrew for "my father's joy," Abigail symbolizes delight and grace, a figure celebrated for wisdom and beauty in the Hebrew Bible. Its timeless appeal reflects kindness and joy, cherished across generations.

- **Alice:** Derived from Germanic *Adalheidis* ("noble"), Alice symbolizes curiosity and resilience. Popularized by *Alice's Adventures in Wonderland*, it combines light elegance with strength, further enriched by figures like Alice Paul and Alice Roosevelt.

- **Brittany:** Of French origin, referring to the region of Brittany, this name gained popularity in the late 20th century. It conveys a sense of modernity and sophistication, with nicknames like Britt adding a playful touch.

- **Claire:** French for "bright" or "clear," Claire conveys purity and elegance. Rooted in the Latin *Clara*, it has a radiant quality, often linked to clarity and light, making it a timeless and refined choice.

- **Clara:** Latin for "bright" and "famous," Clara radiates vintage charm and intelligence. It balances timelessness with modern elegance, making it ideal for parents seeking sophistication.

- **David:** A Hebrew name meaning "beloved," David holds historical and religious significance, often associated with King David's bravery and leadership. Its universal appeal is reflected in variations like Davi (Portuguese) and its cultural symbolism, including the Star of David.

- **Dean:** Derived from the Old English *dene*, meaning "valley," Dean has British roots. Its simplicity and versatility give it lasting charm and adaptability. Often associated with leadership, it's a strong, understated classic.

- **Elise:** A French diminutive of Elizabeth, Elise means "God is my oath." Its soft, graceful sound lends it a refined simplicity. Beloved for its understated elegance, Elise is both classic and contemporary.

- **Ethan:** Hebrew for "strong" or "enduring," Ethan embodies resilience and dependability, with biblical roots tied to wisdom. Its straightforward sound and timeless appeal make it a popular choice worldwide.

- **Grace:** Latin for "favor" or "blessing," Grace embodies kindness, poise, and inner strength. Cherished for its simplicity and elegance, it has roots in virtue names and Greek mythology's Three Graces, with figures like Grace Kelly enhancing its timeless sophistication.

- **Graham:** Of Scottish origin, meaning "gravelly homestead," Graham embodies sophistication and charm. Its timeless appeal makes it a strong, classic choice with a modern edge.

- **Harriet:** Derived from the French name Henriette, Harriet means "home ruler." Popularized by figures like Harriet Tubman, it represents courage and independence. Nicknames like Hattie and Etta bring warmth and charm, blending historical significance with modern appeal.

- **Jack:** Of British origin, Jack means "God is gracious" or "healthy," blending charm and strength. Its Celtic and Old French roots add vitality, making it a classic favorite with enduring energy.

- **Jane:** English for "God is gracious," Jane blends quiet elegance with strength. Celebrated in works like *Jane Eyre* and borne by figures like Jane Austen, it symbolizes resilience and intelligence, balancing warmth with classic appeal.

- **Joel:** Meaning "the Lord is God," Joel originates from Hebrew scripture. Its biblical roots and straightforward sound give it a timeless, grounded quality. Widely used across cultures, Joel is simple yet rich in significance.

- **Julia:** From Latin *Iulius*, Julia means "youthful" or "Jove's child." Its Roman roots and literary connections through Shakespeare and Dickens add to its sophistication and enduring charm, with variants like Juliet and Juliana offering versatility.

- **Justin:** Of Latin origin, meaning "just" or "righteous," Justin symbolizes fairness and virtue. Popular across generations, it maintains a timeless and approachable charm. Justin's simplicity and strength make it universally appealing.

- **Kimberly:** Of Old English origin, meaning "from the wood of the royal fortress," Kimberly rose to popularity in the 20th century. With nicknames like Kim and Kimmie, it blends sophistication with warmth and familiarity.

- **Liam:** An Irish diminutive of William, Liam means "strong-willed warrior" and represents protection and resilience. Its modern charm is complemented by its strong traditional roots, making it universally appealing.

- **Lillian:** Derived from the Latin *lilium*, meaning "lily," Lillian represents purity and renewal. It has Victorian-era charm, with nicknames like Lily and Lillie offering modern versatility. A timeless choice, Lillian conveys elegance while maintaining a warm, approachable feel.

- **Luke:** Derived from Latin *Lucas* ("light-giving"), Luke is associated with Luke the

Evangelist and represents wisdom and kindness. Variants like Luca and Lukas add global adaptability to its modern yet timeless simplicity.

- **Mark:** Latin for "warlike," Mark carries biblical roots with Mark the Evangelist and historical connections to figures like Mark Antony. Known for its simplicity and steady appeal, it reflects strength and quiet confidence.

- **Martha:** Of Aramaic origin, meaning "lady" or "mistress," Martha is known for its simplicity and strength. It has been borne by influential figures like Martha Washington. Nicknames like Marty add a casual touch, balancing tradition with warmth.

- **Molly:** A diminutive of Mary, Molly means "bitter" or "wished-for child" and carries an approachable, cheerful quality. Popular in English-speaking cultures, it has ties to literature and music, adding a playful charm to its enduring appeal.

- **Neil:** Of Irish origin, meaning "champion" or "cloud," Neil is simple yet impactful. Its variants, such as Neal, add versatility, while its understated charm ensures timeless appeal.

- **Owen:** Of Welsh origin, Owen means "noble" or "young warrior." Its enduring popularity stems from its balance of strength and warmth. Widely recognized across cultures, Owen remains a timeless and approachable name.

- **Paul:** Latin for "small" or "humble," Paul is tied to Saint Paul's influence in Christianity. Known for its grounded simplicity, it has been borne by figures like Paul McCartney and Paul Newman, symbolizing humility and strength.

- **Rose:** Latin for "flower," Rose symbolizes beauty, love, and romance, with mythological ties to Aphrodite. Its simplicity and cultural variations like Rosa and Rosalie enhance its delicate, timeless charm.

- **Ruby:** From the Latin *ruber*, meaning "red," Ruby symbolizes passion and vitality, inspired by the precious gemstone. Popularized in the Victorian era, it is a vibrant, nature-inspired name with warmth and energy.

- **Seth:** A Hebrew name meaning "appointed" or "placed," Seth has biblical roots as the third son of Adam and Eve. It carries a calm, grounded quality, making it a strong and approachable name.

- **Troy:** Of Greek origin, Troy refers to the ancient city central to Homer's *Iliad*. Symbolizing heroism and history, it carries a strong and noble appeal. Troy's simplicity and cultural resonance keep it timelessly relevant.

- **Tyler:** Of Old English origin, meaning "maker of tiles," Tyler is a modern classic. Popularized in the 20th century, it has a fresh, approachable vibe and works equally well for boys and girls.

Choosing a simple, classic name ensures that it remains relevant throughout life, embodying qualities of stability and quiet strength.

Cross-Cultural Endurance

Classic names often resonate across cultures, giving them universal appeal. Names like Maria and Daniel feel at home in various languages and traditions, bridging cultural boundaries with ease.

Examples include:

- **Adriana:** Of Latin origin, Adriana means "from Hadria," referring to the Adriatic region. It carries elegance and strength, with historical ties to Roman culture. Adriana's melodic appeal and international adaptability make it enduringly popular.

- **Amelie:** A French variant of Amelia, Amelie means "industrious" or "striving." Its soft, melodic tone and European charm give it a timeless sophistication. Amelie blends classic elegance with a modern, international flair.

- **Anna:** A Hebrew name meaning "grace" or "favor," Anna is cherished for its simplicity and kindness. Variations like Ana, Anya, and Anne add cultural versatility. Associated with Saint Anne and literary icons, Anna maintains its universal charm across generations.

- **Anya:** A Russian diminutive of Anna, Anya means "grace" or "favor." Rooted in Slavic traditions, it carries a sense of elegance and strength. Its cross-cultural charm ensures its lasting popularity and appeal.

- **Arabella:** Derived from Latin and Old English, Arabella means "yielding to prayer" or "beautiful altar." Historically tied to British aristocracy, it conveys sophistication and grace. Its romantic, melodic sound gives it an enduring, classic charm.

- **Carmen:** Of Latin origin, meaning "song" or "poem," Carmen reflects creativity and expression. Its strong ties to Spanish culture and the famous opera *Carmen* enrich its legacy. Carmen's simplicity and depth make it a classic with global appeal.

- **Daniel:** Hebrew for "God is my judge," Daniel symbolizes resilience, intelligence, and integrity, inspired by the biblical figure known for his faith and wisdom. Variations like Danilo and Daniil enhance its global appeal, making Daniel a cherished name worldwide.

- **Giselle:** Of Germanic origin, Giselle means "pledge" or "hostage." Popularized by the iconic ballet *Giselle*, it carries a sense of elegance and artistry. Its international appeal makes it both timeless and culturally versatile.

- **Ingrid:** Of Norse origin, this name means "beautiful" or "beloved." It is tied to

Scandinavian royalty and iconic figures like actress Ingrid Bergman. With its dignified charm, Ingrid remains a timeless name full of strength.

- **Isabella:** A Hebrew-Italian name meaning "devoted to God," Isabella also translates to "beautiful" in Italian. Its royal, literary, and melodic qualities make it a perennial favorite, blending spirituality and beauty with lasting appeal.

- **Jacob:** A Hebrew name meaning "supplanter," Jacob is rooted in the Torah and symbolizes determination and adaptability. Its versatility and presence in literature and modern culture make it a timeless choice, representing strength and individuality.

- **Jasmine:** Derived from the Persian *yasmin*, meaning "gift from God," Jasmine reflects beauty and purity. Inspired by the fragrant flower, it is a timeless name with natural elegance. Popular across cultures, Jasmine's lyrical sound ensures its enduring use.

- **John:** Derived from Hebrew *Yohanan* ("God is gracious"), John is known for its strength, honor, and deep biblical roots. Variations like Juan, Jean, Giovanni, and Ivan reflect its adaptability, making it a universally respected and enduring classic.

- **Maria:** Of Latin origin, Maria means "bitter," "beloved," or "wished-for child." Closely tied to the Virgin Mary, it symbolizes love, faith, and devotion. Widely used across cultures, variations like Marie, Marija, and Mary highlight its global appeal and adaptability, making it a timeless name.

- **Marshall:** An Old French name meaning "caretaker of horses," Marshall reflects strength and tradition. Its bold, commanding sound gives it a timeless, classic appeal. Marshall's versatility and dignified tone make it a strong choice.

- **Naomi:** A Hebrew name meaning "pleasantness" or "delight," Naomi is deeply rooted in biblical tradition. Associated with faith and resilience, it carries significant spiritual weight. Its simplicity and warmth ensure its lasting appeal across generations.

- **Regina:** Latin for "queen," Regina symbolizes authority and grace. Its regal associations and historical significance give it a strong yet approachable feel. Often tied to royalty and saints, Regina is a name of enduring dignity.

- **Sarah:** Meaning "princess" or "noblewoman" in Hebrew, Sarah is celebrated for its strength and biblical significance as the matriarch of the Jewish people. Variants like Sara add to its cross-cultural charm, ensuring its timeless elegance resonates across generations.

- **Silvia:** From the Latin *silva* ("forest"), Silvia evokes natural beauty and serenity. This ancient

Roman name is classic and elegant, carrying a timeless appeal. Its connection to nature and mythology ensures its enduring charm.

- **Vanessa:** Created by Jonathan Swift in his poem *Cadenus and Vanessa*, this name signifies creativity. Its modern associations with charm have ensured its lasting appeal. Vanessa is sophisticated yet approachable, making it a timeless favorite.

These names honor heritage while remaining adaptable, making them ideal for families seeking a connection to multiple cultures or a name that feels universal.

Emotional and Familial Connections

Family-inspired names carry emotional weight, connecting children to their roots. Choosing a name like Edward or Margaret to honor a beloved relative creates a lasting bond between generations, tying your child to the values and stories of their ancestors.

Examples include:

- **Amelia:** Latin for "industrious" or "striving," Amelia emphasizes ambition and integrity. Variants like Amelie add sophistication, making it a versatile name reflecting determination and elegance.

- **Annabelle:** Annabelle combines the Hebrew *Anna* ("grace") with the French *belle* ("beautiful"). This name exudes timeless charm with its melodic sound and versatility. Annabelle is both vintage and modern, offering a balance of grace and warmth.

- **Benjamin:** Hebrew for "son of the right hand," Benjamin is rich in biblical history and emotional depth. Popular nicknames like Ben and Benji add charm, making it a timeless and meaningful choice.

- **Caroline:** With German and French roots meaning "free woman," Caroline blends regal sophistication with approachability. It honors independence and resilience, with versatile nicknames like Carrie and Caro making it a cherished name across generations.

- **Ella:** German for "fairy maiden" or "goddess," Ella exudes grace and lightness, with ties to cultural icons like Ella Fitzgerald, whose musical brilliance adds depth to the name. Rooted in Old English and Germanic traditions, Ella has also been linked to mythology and nobility, making it both timeless and versatile.

- **Edward:** Of Old English origin, meaning "wealthy guardian," Edward symbolizes strength, wisdom, and loyalty. A name borne by kings and saints, it balances formality with friendliness through nicknames like Ed, Eddie, and Ted, making it both dignified and approachable.

- **Evangeline:** Derived from Greek *euangelion* ("good news"), Evangeline symbolizes hope and light. Its literary associations, notably Longfellow's poem *Evangeline*, add romantic depth. With its ethereal quality, Evangeline remains a beloved classic with spiritual ties.

- **Francis:** Latin for "free man," Francis is associated with humility and kindness, inspired by Saint Francis of Assisi. Gender-neutral and globally adaptable, it offers variations like Francisco and Francesca and friendly nicknames like Frank and Frankie.

- **Harold:** Meaning "ruler of the army" in Old English, Harold embodies leadership and tradition. Favored by European royals, it maintains a familiar, warm appeal through nicknames like Harry and Hal, making it a classic name tied to loyalty and strength.

- **Joseph:** A Hebrew name meaning "God will increase," Joseph reflects strength, humility, and family devotion. Popular variants like Joe, Joey, and Giuseppe add warmth, while the feminine Josephine offers elegance and charm with nicknames like Josie and Jo.

- **Madeline:** Of Hebrew origin, meaning "tower" or "from Magdala," Madeline symbolizes strength and steadfastness. Its literary appeal and nostalgic charm come from Ludwig

Bemelmans's beloved *Madeline* series, making it an elegant and enduring choice.

- **Margaret:** Greek for "pearl," Margaret represents purity and resilience. Carried by saints, queens, and leaders like Margaret Thatcher, it combines timeless elegance with versatility, offering nicknames like Maggie, Meg, and Margo.

- **Meredith:** A Welsh name meaning "great ruler" or "sea lord," Meredith reflects strength and leadership. Its gentle sound gives it a refined and approachable quality. Meredith's blend of elegance and versatility makes it a distinguished choice.

- **Penelope:** Of Greek origin, meaning "weaver," Penelope represents loyalty and cleverness, inspired by Homer's *Odyssey*. Associated with grace and resourcefulness, it offers a modern touch with nicknames like Penny, blending tradition with elegance.

- **Samuel:** Hebrew for "God has heard," Samuel is a biblically significant name tied to wisdom, faith, and integrity. Its timeless appeal is enhanced by approachable nicknames like Sam and Sammy, making it a beloved classic.

- **Wallace:** Of Old French origin, meaning "foreigner" or "Welshman," Wallace exudes strength and heritage. It reflects a dignified and vintage charm tied to figures like William

Wallace. Wallace's bold and timeless tone makes it a classic option.

These names are just a few examples of how classic names can carry emotional and familial significance. Each family has unique traditions, stories, and names that hold special meaning, and what's cherished in one family may differ in another. That's the beauty of family-inspired names—they're deeply personal choices that connect to the heart and history of your specific family.

Wrapping Up

Classic names like Elizabeth, William, and Grace offer more than just elegance—they are timeless gifts that bridge the past and the present. Whether chosen for their simplicity, cultural resonance, or familial significance, these names carry grace and strength across generations.

As you reflect on these enduring choices, consider what resonates most with your family's story. In the next chapter, we'll explore rare and unique names for parents seeking individuality and modern appeal—names that offer a fresh perspective on your child's legacy.

Chapter 3:
Unique and Rare Baby Names

When it comes to naming your child, choosing something unique and rare can be incredibly exciting—and meaningful. While classic names have their timeless charm, there's something special about giving your child a name that feels one of a kind—a name that stands apart and reflects your hopes and dreams for them. In this chapter, we'll explore rare and unique names that offer both personality and purpose, helping you find the perfect choice for your child.

Unique names go beyond simply being different; they carry hidden meanings, cultural ties, and qualities that reflect a life of courage, kindness, or creativity. These names ensure that your child's identity feels truly their own, free from the commonality of more popular names. Whether you're drawn to modern, uncommon choices or the revival of rare gems from history, this chapter offers inspiration for names that are as distinctive as they are meaningful.

The Appeal of Unique Names

Unique names have an undeniable charm, providing a way to celebrate what makes your child special. These names often carry a sense of individuality, ensuring your child's name stands out in any setting. In a world where trends come and go, unique names offer stability, serving as a lasting marker of your child's personality and heritage.

For many parents, the allure of unique names lies in their originality and the opportunity to express meaningful qualities. A rare name can reflect your dreams for your child, connecting them to values or cultural roots while ensuring they carry a name that feels fresh and innovative.

Here are some examples:

- **Alden:** An Old English name meaning "old friend," Alden conveys warmth, loyalty, and sage wisdom. Its gentle, timeless appeal makes it a thoughtful choice for parents who value enduring companionship and reliability.

- **Alora:** From the Bantu language of Botswana, Alora means "my dream," reflecting aspiration and hope. Also tied to Latin *laurus* ("laurel tree"), it symbolizes victory and growth, offering a name that is both graceful and meaningful.

- **Atlas:** A bold Greek name meaning "to carry" or "endure," Atlas is tied to the mythological Titan who held up the sky. Symbolizing resilience and exploration, it conveys strength and worldliness, offering a powerful choice for adventurous spirits.

- **Azura:** From Old Persian, Azura means "sky blue," evoking the vastness and serenity of the sky. Symbolizing peace and natural beauty, this ethereal name offers modern grace with a timeless connection to nature.

- **Benson:** An English surname meaning "son of Ben," Benson exudes a strong yet friendly charm. Its modern feel and versatile sound make it suitable for any gender. Benson is both unique and accessible, offering a contemporary edge.

- **Calix:** Originating from Greek *kállistos* ("very handsome" or "wonderful"), Calix blends classical elegance with a modern touch. Its meaning ties to beauty and allure, making it a sophisticated yet unique choice for parents seeking charm and charisma.

- **Dalton:** An Old English name meaning "valley town," Dalton evokes a rustic charm. Its steady and strong sound gives it a timeless, unique quality. It offers a balance of tradition and individuality.

- **Dashiell:** A French surname with an uncertain origin, Dashiell conveys sophistication and modern flair. Often associated with the author Dashiell Hammett, it suggests creativity, wit, and individuality, with a distinctive sound that makes it memorable.

- **Desmond:** Of Irish origin, meaning "from South Munster," Desmond carries a refined yet rugged appeal. Its historical significance is complemented by its modern versatility. Desmond's timeless charm makes it a distinctive unisex option.

- **Draven:** Of modern origin, Draven is associated with strength and mystery, often linked to the concept of bravery. Its edgy and distinctive sound makes it a bold choice for parents seeking something unconventional yet striking.

- **Griffin:** Of Welsh and Irish origin, Griffin means "lord" or "prince" and is inspired by the mythical lion-eagle creature. Representing courage, strength, and wisdom, it carries a noble, mystical essence with a modern, approachable edge.

- **Kayden:** A modern name with Celtic and American roots, Kayden means "fighter" or "companion." Its sleek, modern sound gives it a bold and versatile appeal. Kayden's rising popularity reflects its contemporary charm.

- **Maisie:** A Scottish diminutive of Margaret, Maisie means "pearl." Playful and charming, it has a vintage feel with a modern resurgence. Its rarity adds a touch of whimsy to its timeless appeal.

- **Mireille:** A French name meaning "to admire" or "to look," Mireille exudes elegance and charm. Its melodic quality and positive connotations make it a sophisticated yet heartfelt option, ideal for those seeking a name with grace and beauty.

- **Oberon:** Derived from Germanic origins, Oberon means "noble bear" or "king of the fairies." Popularized by Shakespeare's *A Midsummer Night's Dream,* it embodies magic, strength, and nobility, with Obi as a playful nickname.

- **Orson:** Of Latin origin, meaning "bear," Orson conveys strength and courage. Its rare, vintage charm gives it a distinctive and memorable quality. Orson's rugged yet approachable tone ensures its timeless appeal.

- **Quentin:** A Latin name meaning "fifth," Quentin is associated with order and creativity. Its modern usage gives it a refined yet edgy appeal. Quentin's distinctive sound and versatility make it a stylish, timeless choice.

- **Quinley:** An English name meaning "estate of the queen," Quinley offers a regal yet playful feel. Its blend of traditional roots and modern style makes it a versatile choice for parents seeking something fresh and distinctive.

- **Ryder:** Of Old English origin, Ryder means "mounted warrior" or "messenger." It exudes adventure and strength, giving it a modern, edgy appeal. Unique yet recognizable, Ryder is ideal for a bold and active personality.

- **Ryker:** Derived from Dutch origins, Ryker means "rich" or "powerful." This bold, modern name exudes strength and resilience, making it a dynamic choice for parents seeking a name with a commanding presence.

- **Waverly:** An English name meaning "meadow of quivering aspens," Waverly evokes a sense of nature's beauty and tranquility. With its melodic sound, it offers a whimsical yet grounded choice for parents who value a connection to the outdoors.

- **Xander:** A short form of Alexander, Xander means "defender of the people." This Greek-derived name is vibrant and modern while maintaining its connection to a strong and noble legacy.

- **Zoey:** A Greek name meaning "life," Zoey is vibrant and full of energy. Its modern spelling adds a fresh, unique twist to a timeless classic. With its playful tone, Zoey exudes charm and individuality.

Choosing a unique name is more than just finding something rare—it's about giving your child a name that reflects qualities you value and the stories you wish to share. Unique names offer the chance to set your child's identity apart, creating a legacy of individuality and meaning that will stay with them throughout life.

Balancing Uniqueness With Practicality

While the appeal of unique names is undeniable, it's important to consider usability. A unique name that is also easy to pronounce and spell offers the perfect balance, ensuring it remains memorable without causing confusion. Practical names with distinctive qualities allow your child to carry a name that feels both special and approachable in daily life.

A practical yet rare name is a meaningful choice for parents who want to avoid overly complicated spellings or pronunciations. These names maintain a sense of individuality while being simple enough to navigate both personal and professional settings.

Some examples might include:

- **Andre:** The French and Portuguese form of Andrew, meaning "manly" or "brave." Andre's smooth, sophisticated sound gives it a modern yet timeless feel. Its multicultural appeal ensures its relevance across generations and regions.

- **Beckett:** An English surname meaning "bee cottage," Beckett has a literary connection through playwright Samuel Beckett. It embodies intellect, resilience, and charm, offering a stylish and contemporary feel.

- **Brynn:** A Welsh name meaning "hill," Brynn is simple yet distinctive. Its soft sound makes it approachable, while its rarity ensures individuality. It blends nature-inspired charm with a sleek, modern feel.

- **Cassia:** Derived from Greek and Latin origins, Cassia means "cinnamon," symbolizing spice and warmth. This exotic yet familiar name carries an elegant simplicity, perfect for parents who want a name with both charm and depth.

- **Cleo:** Derived from Greek, Cleo means "glory" or "pride." As a diminutive of Cleopatra, it carries regal history and vibrant simplicity, offering a memorable, approachable option.

- **Corbin:** From Old French and Latin, Corbin means "raven" or "crow." Symbolizing intelligence and mystery, this sleek name is linked to nature and has a modern yet grounded appeal, perfect for parents seeking something unique but not outlandish.

- **Dax:** From French and Latin origins, Dax means "leader" or "water." This succinct, modern name also refers to the French spa town known for its healing waters. With its contemporary appeal, Dax is a bold yet practical choice.

- **Esme:** Of French origin, meaning "esteemed" or "loved," Esme offers elegance and simplicity. Linked to Esmeralda ("emerald"), it evokes value and beauty, making it both sophisticated and memorable.

- **Faye:** A name of English, French, and Latin origins, Faye means "fairy," "belief," and "loyalty." Its mystical charm and elegance evoke trust and whimsy, making it a versatile choice.

- **Flint:** An English name meaning "hard stone," Flint symbolizes resilience and durability. Its short, strong sound gives it a modern, edgy vibe. Rarely used, Flint stands out as a bold and unique choice.

- **Holden:** Meaning "hollow valley," Holden originates from Old English. Popularized by *The Catcher in the Rye*, it carries literary sophistication. Its modern rarity paired with vintage roots makes it uniquely appealing.

- **Homer:** Of Greek origin, Homer means "pledge" or "hostage." It is famously tied to the ancient poet of *Iliad* and *Odyssey*, symbolizing intellect and creativity. Homer's literary roots give it a timeless and scholarly appeal.

- **Ivo:** A Germanic and Hebrew name meaning "yew tree" or "God is gracious," Ivo represents resilience and divine grace. Compact and grounded, it balances strength with accessibility.

- **Ivy:** An English name symbolizing fidelity and friendship, Ivy is inspired by the evergreen climbing plant. Simple yet unique, it combines a timeless, gentle sound with natural elegance.

- **Keanu:** Of Hawaiian origin, meaning "cool breeze over the mountains," Keanu exudes calm and strength. It carries a serene and natural tone, popularized by actor Keanu Reeves. Keanu's cultural depth and unique sound make it a standout choice.

- **Kieran:** An Irish name meaning "little dark one," Kieran blends tradition and modernity. Associated with Saint Ciarán of Clonmacnoise, it conveys cultural depth and approachability.

- **Mira:** With Latin, Slavic, and Sanskrit roots, Mira means "admirable," "peace," and "ocean." This multicultural name has literary ties, appearing in works like Shakespeare's *The Tempest*, and is celebrated for its universal appeal.

- **Nia:** Rooted in Swahili, Welsh, and Irish traditions, Nia means "purpose," "aim," or "goal" in Swahili and "bright" in Welsh. Rich in cultural significance, it embodies clarity, unity, and intention.

- **Otis:** With German origins, meaning "wealth" or "prosperity," Otis combines vintage charm with simplicity. Its straightforward sound has a timeless appeal.

- **Piper:** Of English origin, Piper means "flute player." This musical name feels fresh and modern, with a lively, cheerful energy. Its unique sound ensures it stands out without feeling overly trendy.

- **Porter:** An English occupational name meaning "gatekeeper," Porter conveys dependability and a grounded nature. Its polished yet approachable sound makes it a stylish choice for parents drawn to surname-inspired names.

- **Ross:** A name of Scottish and Old Norse origin, meaning "headland" or "promontory." Ross reflects strength and nature, with a sleek, modern tone. Its short, straightforward sound makes it versatile and timeless.

- **Sienna:** Derived from the Italian city known for its reddish-brown clay, Sienna symbolizes warmth and artistic beauty. This name reflects a love of nature and culture, making it an elegant and vibrant choice.

- **Soren:** A Scandinavian name derived from Latin *severus* ("stern" or "strict"), Soren reflects strength and depth. Its intellectual yet approachable tone is tied to philosopher Søren Kierkegaard.

- **Tobin:** Of Hebrew origin, Tobin means "God is good." A rare and friendly name, it carries a sense of kindness and warmth, offering a fresh alternative to more traditional names like Tobias.

- **Vlad:** Of Slavic origin, Vlad means "rule" or "power." It is tied to historical figures like Vlad the Impaler, adding a bold, mysterious quality. Vlad's strong and striking tone makes it a distinctive choice.

- **Zuri:** With Swahili and Basque origins, Zuri means "beautiful" or "white." This name evokes a sense of purity and connection to nature, often associated with joy and elegance. Its simplicity and cultural depth make it a fresh and radiant choice.

Choosing a unique yet practical name lets you give your child an identity that is both special and approachable. It allows your child to navigate both personal and professional settings with a name that feels distinctive yet accessible.

Rare Names With a Cultural and Global Perspective

Names with global roots bring cultural richness and diversity to your child's identity. These names are often deeply tied to traditions, histories, and values from around the world, offering a meaningful way to honor heritage while still choosing something rare. A name with cultural significance can connect your child to a sense of belonging while standing out for its unique beauty.

For example:

- **Aarav:** A Sanskrit name meaning "peaceful" or "melodious." Aarav's calming tone and spiritual roots make it a unique choice. Its growing popularity reflects its modern yet meaningful essence.

- **Alissa:** A name with German and Arabic roots, Alissa means "nobility" or "wanderer." It combines grace with curiosity and offers flexible variants like Alyssa and Larissa, adding versatility to its charm.

- **Amara:** A multicultural name with Igbo and Latin roots, Amara means "grace" and "immortal." It reflects beauty, resilience, and kindness, resonating across cultures with timeless charm.

- **Ananya:** A Sanskrit name meaning "unique" or "incomparable," Ananya exudes elegance and spiritual significance, reflecting individuality. Its lyrical sound ensures its rarity and appeal in a global context.

- **Ari:** With Hebrew, Norse, and Armenian origins, Ari means "lion" (Hebrew) and "eagle" (Norse), symbolizing strength, bravery, and freedom. This short and powerful name is bold yet approachable, ideal for parents seeking simplicity and resilience.

- **Arwen:** With Welsh origins, Arwen means "noble maiden" or "muse." Known from Tolkien's *The Lord of the Rings*, it embodies grace, bravery, and lyrical beauty, perfect for parents valuing heritage and mythology.

- **Astrid:** Of Scandinavian origin, Astrid means "divine strength" or "godly beauty." This elegant name carries an air of royalty and grace, making it an inspiring choice for parents drawn to Nordic heritage and powerful femininity.

- **August:** With Latin origins, meaning "great" or "majestic," August is linked to Emperor Augustus and symbolizes leadership and respect. Its dignified yet gentle nature is versatile across cultures.

- **Brielle:** A diminutive of Gabrielle, Brielle means "God is my strength." Its soft, melodic sound and rarity make it a distinctive and feminine choice. It blends biblical roots with modern appeal.

- **Cyrus:** A Persian name meaning "sun" or "lord," Cyrus is associated with the ancient king Cyrus the Great, symbolizing wisdom and vitality. Its regal and life-affirming qualities make it a strong, luminous choice.

- **Declan:** Of Irish origin, Declan means "man of prayer" or "full of goodness." Rooted in Gaelic tradition, it carries a strong, spiritual resonance. Its unique sound and heritage ensure its enduring appeal.

- **Egal:** Derived from Somali origins, Egal means "equal" or "justice." This rare and meaningful name carries a sense of balance and fairness, perfect for parents drawn to its empowering and unique qualities.

- **Emil:** Derived from the Latin *Aemilius*, Emil means "rival" or "eager." This name has a refined simplicity, making it rare yet approachable. Its European flair adds a cosmopolitan touch to its charm.

- **Finnegan:** Of Irish origin, Finnegan means "white" or "fair-haired" and is tied to Irish mythology and literary heritage. Shortened to Finn, it balances cultural roots with modern appeal.

- **Kade:** A modern variation of Cade, meaning "round" or "barrel," Kade feels sleek and contemporary. Its short, strong sound gives it a bold yet approachable vibe. Rare and versatile, Kade suits those seeking a fresh, distinctive name.

- **Kenzo:** Of Japanese origin, Kenzo means "strong and healthy." This stylish and unique name carries a sense of energy and resilience, ideal for parents who value strength and creativity.

- **Levent:** A Turkish and Greek name meaning "handsome" or "strong," Levent has noble historical ties, particularly among Ottoman sailors. Its cosmopolitan flair and strength make it a distinguished choice.

- **Malcolm:** Of Scottish origin, Malcolm means "disciple of Saint Columba." It carries a regal and historical weight, paired with a modern edge. This strong, rare name exudes intelligence and leadership.

- **Marisol:** Combining "sea" and "sun" in Spanish, Marisol evokes natural beauty and warmth. This poetic name is ideal for parents drawn to imagery of nature and a sense of place.

- **Mika:** A name with Japanese and Hebrew origins, Mika means "new moon" or "who is like God." Its gentle, melodic sound adds to its unique and serene charm. Mika's cross-cultural versatility makes it a rare yet adaptable choice.

- **Niall:** Of Irish origin, Niall means "champion" or "cloud." This ancient name carries a sense of strength and mystery, blending a rich cultural history with modern appeal.

- **Nilo:** A Spanish and Egyptian name referring to the Nile River, Nilo symbolizes life and prosperity. It honors ancient heritage while offering a contemporary, refreshing appeal.

- **Nina:** A multicultural name with Native American, Spanish, Slavic, and Hindi roots, Nina means "little girl" (Spanish), "fire" (Quechua), "grace" (Slavic), and "beautiful eyes" (Hindi). Its warmth and versatility make it a lovely choice that celebrates beauty and heritage.

- **Noel:** Of French and Latin origin, Noel means "Christmas" or "born on Christmas." It reflects joy, togetherness, and timeless elegance, suitable for all seasons and cultures.

- **Otto:** Of German origin, Otto means "wealth" or "prosperity." With deep royal and historical connections, this name has been borne by kings and leaders, blending tradition with a contemporary edge.

- **Paloma:** Of Spanish origin, Paloma means "dove," a symbol of peace and love. This graceful name carries a soft yet powerful connotation, ideal for parents who value serenity and compassion.

- **Pax:** Of Latin origin, Pax means "peace." Linked to the Roman goddess of peace, it symbolizes harmony, unity, and tranquility, making it a serene and meaningful choice.

- **Roman:** Meaning "citizen of Rome," Roman has a strong historical resonance. With its bold sound, it feels modern while carrying ancient roots. Its international usage adds to its rare yet familiar appeal.

- **Saskia:** Of Dutch and German origin, Saskia means "protector of mankind." This name has historical significance, as it is tied to Dutch nobility and the arts, notably through Rembrandt's wife Saskia van Uylenburgh, making it culturally significant.

- **Soraya:** Of Persian origin, Soraya means "jewel" or "the Pleiades," referencing a cluster of stars. This celestial name embodies grace, beauty, and mystery, making it ideal for parents who love names with cosmic resonance.

- **Tove:** Of Scandinavian origin, Tove means "beautiful" or "peace." A short yet impactful name, Tove blends simplicity with strength, offering a timeless Nordic charm that feels both ancient and modern.

- **Yasmin:** Of Persian origin, Yasmin means "jasmine flower," symbolizing beauty, grace, and love. A timeless and fragrant choice, it resonates across cultures and carries a gentle, sophisticated charm.

- **Zara:** Of Arabic and Hebrew origins, Zara means "blooming flower" or "princess." With its sleek, modern feel, it is both sophisticated and globally resonant. Zara's rarity paired with its regal tone ensures a distinctive appeal.

These names embody cultural richness and individuality, fostering a sense of belonging, strength, and a deep connection between personal identity and global heritage.

Uncommon Names With Deep Meanings

For parents who want a name that reflects values or ideals, uncommon names with profound meanings are a perfect choice. These names go beyond being rare; they carry a story, often symbolizing qualities like resilience, love, or creativity. A meaningful name becomes a gift, inspiring your child throughout their life.

Examples include:

- **Acacia:** From Greek origins, Acacia refers to the resilient and thorny tree, symbolizing strength and immortality. This nature-inspired name is both rare and timeless, making it ideal for parents drawn to its botanical beauty.

- **Adair:** Of Scottish origin, Adair means "oak tree ford." This nature-inspired name is rare and sophisticated, exuding quiet strength. Its historical roots and contemporary edge give it lasting appeal.

- **Amias:** With Latin and French origins, Amias means "beloved" and conveys love, compassion, and kindness. This warm, gentle name inspires meaningful connections, offering a distinctive yet accessible charm.

- **Arlette:** Of French origin, Arlette means "noble" or "little eagle." This name exudes sophistication and strength, combining a sense of tradition with a fresh, stylish sound.

- **Carver:** Derived from the Old English word for "sculptor" or "carpenter," Carver symbolizes creativity and craftsmanship. This strong, earthy name is perfect for parents who value artistry and practicality.

- **Cassidy:** An Irish name meaning "clever" or "curly-haired," Cassidy has a playful appeal. Its versatility makes it suitable for both genders, adding to its uniqueness. With its upbeat sound, Cassidy feels both friendly and rare.

- **Cedric:** Of Celtic origin, Cedric means "bounty" or "kindly." Popularized by Sir Walter Scott's *Ivanhoe*, it evokes a sense of history, nobility, and warmth, offering a refined yet approachable choice.

- **Clover:** An English name symbolizing luck and abundance, Clover evokes images of greenery and charm. Its whimsical yet grounded feel makes it an appealing option for parents who love names connected to nature and positivity.

- **Colson:** A name of English origin, Colson means "son of Nicholas." This contemporary-sounding name offers a blend of traditional roots and modern appeal, making it ideal for parents who value heritage with a fresh twist.

- **Colton:** An Old English name meaning "coal town," Colton reflects ruggedness and strength. Modern and versatile, it carries a cool, distinctive vibe. Its connection to nature and industry makes it uniquely appealing.

- **Darius:** With Persian origins, Darius means "possessor of good" or "kingly." A strong, regal name, Darius is associated with ancient Persian rulers, symbolizing leadership, wisdom, and strength.

- **Daya:** With Sanskrit and Hebrew roots, Daya means "compassion" or "bird of prey." This name balances strength and kindness, offering a versatile and meaningful choice for parents seeking something both gentle and powerful.

- **Delaney:** Of Irish origin, Delaney means "descendant of the challenger." It carries a lively, modern feel while retaining its Gaelic roots. Its unique yet approachable quality makes it a standout choice.

- **Dion:** Of Greek origin, Dion is derived from *Dionysius*, meaning "follower of Dionysus," the god of wine and revelry. A strong yet approachable name, Dion carries a sense of creativity and celebration, perfect for a child with a spirited personality.

- **Eldon:** Derived from Old English, Eldon means "old hill." This rare name reflects steadiness and a connection to nature, making it an appealing option for parents seeking a name that combines rustic charm with enduring simplicity.

- **Emberly:** A modern name derived from "ember," Emberly symbolizes warmth, light, and passion. Its melodic sound and natural imagery make it a glowing choice for parents seeking a name with both contemporary appeal and a touch of nature.

- **Enoch:** Of Hebrew origin, Enoch means "dedicated" or "devoted." A biblical name, Enoch was a figure known for his righteousness and closeness to God. This timeless name conveys devotion and spiritual strength, offering a meaningful choice with deep roots in tradition.

- **Evie:** A diminutive of Eva, Evelyn, or Evangeline, Evie means "life" or "living" in Hebrew and Latin. This sweet, lighthearted name reflects vitality, curiosity, and a joyful embrace of new beginnings.

- **Galadriel:** Inspired by Tolkien's *The Lord of the Rings*, Galadriel means "maiden crowned with a radiant garland" in Sindarin Elvish. It embodies beauty, grace, and literary charm, perfect for parents drawn to ethereal and magical qualities.

- **Gideon:** Of Hebrew origin, Gideon means "mighty warrior." A biblical name with deep roots, Gideon embodies strength, faith, and resilience, making it a powerful and timeless choice for parents drawn to meaningful tradition.

- **Hania:** A name of Arabic and Hebrew origins, Hania means "happiness" or "grace." It carries a soft, uplifting tone, symbolizing joy and serenity. Its cultural richness and gentle sound make it an uncommon gem.

- **Harlan:** Of Old English origin, Harlan means "rocky land." This rugged yet modern name evokes a sense of strength and connection to nature, offering a timeless choice for parents seeking a name with a solid foundation.

- **Imara:** From Swahili roots, Imara means "strong" or "steadfast." This powerful name embodies courage, resilience, and determination, ideal for parents who value strength and grace.

- **Indigo:** A name inspired by the deep blue dye, Indigo reflects creativity and individuality. It exudes a sense of mystery and depth, tied to both nature and artistry. Its rare usage ensures a standout, vibrant choice.

- **Katura:** Of Hebrew origin, Katura means "crown" or "encircled." This elegant and rare name evokes a sense of royalty and timeless grace, offering a distinctive choice for parents drawn to its meaningful heritage.

- **Kavi:** Of Indian origin, Kavi means "wise poet," symbolizing creativity and intellectual depth. Rooted in Indian poetry, it encourages artistic expression and a visionary perspective, making it a meaningful choice for parents seeking wisdom and uniqueness.

- **Lucien:** Of French and Latin origins, Lucien means "light." This refined and sophisticated name exudes elegance and intellect, perfect for parents seeking a timeless yet distinctive choice.

- **Myra:** Derived from Greek and Latin origins, Myra means "myrrh," an aromatic resin associated with healing and spirituality. This gentle name carries a timeless elegance, symbolizing compassion and inner strength.

- **Noemi:** A name of Hebrew origin, Noemi means "pleasantness" or "delight." Popular in various cultures, including Spanish and Italian traditions, it exudes warmth and charm, making it a versatile and heartfelt choice.

- **Rafferty:** An Irish name meaning "prosperity wielder" or "flood tide," Rafferty exudes energy and positivity. Its rhythmic charm and playful nicknames like Raff or Rafe make it a lively yet grounded choice.

- **Riona:** Of Irish origin, Riona means "queenly" or "pure." Its lyrical and elegant tone adds a regal quality to its rarity. With deep Gaelic roots, Riona feels both timeless and unique.

- **Simone:** A French name derived from Hebrew *Shimon*, meaning "one who hears," Simone combines elegance with a modern, sophisticated edge. Its rarity and cultural versatility make it a standout choice.

- **Tristan:** Of Celtic origin, Tristan means "sorrowful" or "tumult." Popularized by the Arthurian legend *Tristan and Isolde*, it carries a romantic and adventurous spirit, perfect for parents drawn to literary and historical connections.

- **Vesper:** Latin for "evening star" or "evening prayer," Vesper evokes tranquility and celestial beauty. Its connection to the evening sky and mystical qualities makes it ideal for parents seeking a gentle, luminous name.

- **Zaira:** Of Arabic origin, Zaira means "brightness" or "blooming flower." This radiant name symbolizes growth, light, and resilience, offering a versatile choice that resonates with beauty across languages.

- **Zane:** Of Hebrew origin, Zane means "God is gracious." A sleek, modern name with timeless roots, Zane offers simplicity and strength, making it a versatile choice for parents seeking a bold yet approachable option.

Each of these names embodies both uniqueness and profound meaning, reflecting the qualities parents hope to instill in their children. They add a sense of purpose and identity to a child's life, creating a meaningful legacy to inspire them as they grow.

Wrapping Up

As we conclude this chapter on unique and rare names, we hope you've discovered how these distinct choices can celebrate individuality and meaning in ways that truly stand out. From cultural connections to deep-rooted meanings, these names bring both freshness and a timeless appeal that lasts through life.

For those drawn to names that capture the magic of the world around us, we'll next dive into the beauty of nature-inspired and mythological names. The next chapter will explore names rooted in the earth, sky, and ancient tales, perfect for parents looking to instill a sense of wonder and connection to the natural and mythical world.

Chapter 4:
Nature-Inspired and Mythological Names

In a world increasingly captivated by the beauty and strength of the natural world, many parents are drawn to names that connect their children to the elements and stories that have inspired humanity for centuries. This chapter offers a selection that celebrates the majesty of nature and the powerful resonance of mythology, grounding each name in symbolism and significance. After exploring timeless classics and rare, distinctive names in earlier chapters, we now turn to names that carry a sense of wonder, balance, and heritage that only nature and mythology can provide.

Nature-inspired names evoke grounding, peace, and connection to the earth, sky, water, and fire. From the simplicity of Lily to the uniqueness of Zephyr, they embody qualities like resilience, freedom, and renewal. Mythological names, rich in history and mystery, offer ties to gods, goddesses, and heroes, linking children to virtues like courage, wisdom, and creativity. Names like Athena and Apollo carry stories of wisdom and strength, blending legendary appeal with modern significance.

Let's explore names that echo the majesty of nature and the wisdom of mythology, creating a meaningful choice for your child's lifelong journey!

The Appeal of Nature-Inspired Names

Choosing a nature-inspired name creates a deep connection to the world's natural beauty, resilience, and tranquility. These names capture the essence of landscapes, plants, and peaceful settings, embodying qualities like strength, harmony, and vitality. Many parents seek to instill a sense of grounding and appreciation for the environment, making nature-inspired names a timeless way to connect with these values. They offer many meanings, reminding both the child and family of the qualities they cherish—beauty, growth, resilience, and peace.

Here are some names inspired by nature, each carrying its own story and values to inspire a lifetime.

- **Aspen:** A gender-neutral name of British origin, Aspen means "aspen tree" or "shaking tree." Inspired by the shimmering leaves of the tree, it symbolizes resilience, adaptability, and transformation, evoking the elegance of scenic landscapes.

- **Azalea:** Of Greek origin, meaning "dry," Azalea draws inspiration from the vibrant flowering shrub known for thriving in challenging conditions. Symbolizing resilience and beauty, it reflects strength and elegance, admired for flourishing against the odds.

- **Briar:** Of British origin, meaning "thorny bush of wild roses," Briar represents resilience and balance—beauty paired with strength. Gender-neutral and unique, it's perfect for those who value nature's enduring lessons.

- **Cedar:** A gender-neutral name of Latin and Greek origins, Cedar celebrates the majestic tree known for strength and longevity. Revered in mythology and sacred traditions, it embodies protection and enduring connection to nature.

- **Coral:** Rooted in Latin and Greek origins, Coral reflects the vibrant beauty and resilience of ocean life. Inspired by the intricate structures of coral reefs, this name celebrates strength, natural wonder, and the mysteries of the sea.

- **Cypress:** A gender-neutral name, Cypress is inspired by the resilient cypress tree, representing endurance, protection, and hope. Its elegant quality connects to life's continuity and the enduring strength found in nature.

- **Dahlia:** A flower name of Scandinavian origin, it symbolizes elegance and creativity. The vibrant blooms of the dahlia reflect beauty, strength, and individuality. Its rare and sophisticated tone makes it a standout nature-inspired name.

- **Daisy:** A flower name of Old English origin, Daisy symbolizes purity and innocence. Its cheerful and timeless quality makes it a perennial favorite. Daisy's simplicity and connection to nature give it a fresh, vibrant appeal.

- **Dawn:** A British-origin name symbolizing the first light of day, Dawn signifies new beginnings and hope. Its poetic and radiant quality makes it an inspiring choice for a child who brings light and renewal.

- **Elowen:** Of Cornish origin, Elowen means "elm tree" and represents growth, stability, and grace. This elegant, melodic name feels both modern and timeless, perfect for celebrating nature's beauty and resilience.

- **Fern:** Rooted in Old English, Fern represents humility, sincerity, and eternal life. This enduring name pays homage to the ancient and mysterious plant, a quiet symbol of resilience and timeless elegance.

- **Iris:** Of Greek origin, meaning "rainbow," Iris symbolizes beauty, hope, and individuality. Linked to the delicate flower and the Greek goddess of the rainbow, this elegant name conveys ethereal charm and uniqueness.

- **Isla:** Of Scottish origin, Isla means "island," reflecting tranquility and natural beauty. Its simple yet elegant sound gives it a modern yet classic feel. Rooted in nature, Isla captures serenity and charm.

- **Jade:** Of British origin, meaning "precious stone," Jade symbolizes beauty, prosperity, and wisdom. Associated with protection and healing properties, it blends sophistication with a natural, grounded elegance.

- **Juniper:** Derived from Latin, meaning "evergreen," Juniper reflects vitality, growth, and connection to nature. Known for its aromatic and medicinal properties, this lively name embodies resilience and abundance.

- **Leilani:** A Hawaiian name meaning "heavenly garland of flowers," Leilani is lush and poetic. It symbolizes beauty, grace, and a connection to the earth. Leilani's cultural depth and lyrical tone make it a standout choice.

- **Lily:** Of Latin origin, Lily means "lily flower" or "pure" and symbolizes innocence, grace, and renewal. This versatile name is cherished for its timeless appeal, often used as a standalone or as a pet form of names like Lillian or Elizabeth.

- **Magnolia:** Of French origin, Magnolia is inspired by the magnolia tree, known for its fragrant blossoms symbolizing resilience and elegance. This distinctive name carries Southern charm and natural grace, perfect for celebrating beauty and strength.

- **Meadow:** A name of British and American origin, Meadow evokes pastoral serenity and natural beauty. Conjuring images of open fields and wildflowers, it offers a whimsical yet grounded choice for nature lovers.

- **Mia:** A name of diverse origins—Australian, Latin, and Scandinavian—Mia means "moon," "beloved," and "mine." It evokes nature's grounding, oceanic beauty, and affection, making it a simple yet profoundly meaningful choice.

- **Oliver:** A Latin name meaning "olive tree" or "olive tree planter," Oliver represents peace, dignity, and friendship. Its timeless appeal is enhanced by literary connections like *Oliver Twist* and its rich cultural history.

- **Poppy:** Of Latin and British origins, Poppy is a floral name symbolizing peace, sleep, and remembrance. Its cheerful charm and depth make it a timeless favorite for parents seeking a vivid, nature-inspired name.

- **Raven:** A British name inspired by the intelligent black bird, Raven evokes mystery and individuality. Steeped in literature and folklore, it offers a dramatic flair and a bold choice for a striking personality.

- **Reed:** A nature name referring to the slender, flexible plant, Reed symbolizes adaptability. Its simple and clean sound makes it both modern and classic. Reed's ties to nature and calm energy give it a serene and rare quality.

- **Sage:** An English name of Latin origin, meaning "wise" or "prophet," Sage honors intellect and clarity. This gender-neutral name draws from the aromatic herb and ancient wisdom, adding depth and timeless appeal.

- **Sky:** With English and Scandinavian roots, Sky symbolizes freedom and vast potential. Derived from Old Norse *ský*, meaning "cloud," this gender-neutral name evokes dreams, open possibilities, and the inspiring vastness of the heavens.

- **Sol:** Of Latin origin, meaning "sun," Sol radiates warmth and vitality. Tied to celestial imagery, it symbolizes light and life. Sol's brevity and powerful meaning make it a unique, nature-inspired name.

- **Summer:** Evoking warmth, joy, and vitality, Summer reflects the beauty of the season. This name carries a bright, uplifting tone with timeless appeal. Its connection to nature and positivity ensures its enduring charm.

- **Sylvan:** Derived from the Latin Silvanus, meaning "of the forest," Sylvan evokes ancient groves and serene landscapes. This name symbolizes harmony with nature, offering a peaceful yet adventurous spirit.

- **Violet:** Of Latin origin, Violet means "purple" and is inspired by the delicate violet flower. Popular since the Victorian era, it offers a romantic, timeless charm, complementing other floral classics like Rose and Lily.

- **Willow:** A British-origin name derived from *welig*, meaning "willow tree," Willow symbolizes adaptability, renewal, and quiet strength. Its poetic connection to serene landscapes makes it a timeless tribute to resilience and vitality.

Each of these nature-inspired names offers profound qualities that reflect the values and aspirations parents may have for their child. Whether it's the graceful simplicity of Lily, the quiet strength of Aspen, or the serene mystery of Cypress, nature-inspired names create a meaningful connection to the world's wonders, offering children a timeless identity grounded in the beauty of our natural surroundings.

Names Rooted in the Elements: Earth, Air, Fire, and Water

Choosing a name rooted in the elements—earth, air, fire, and water—offers a powerful connection to the natural forces that sustain life. Each element symbolizes unique qualities, from strength and growth to freedom, passion, and adaptability. Elemental names carry a sense of balance, reflecting the ancient wisdom that nature, in its various forms, holds the power to nurture and protect. For parents drawn to these timeless forces, an elemental name is a beautiful way to give your child a foundation grounded in nature's enduring qualities.

Here are names inspired by earth, air, fire, and water, each with deep meanings and a story to tell.

- **Aeron:** Of Welsh origin, Aeron combines meanings of "berry" and "battle," symbolizing gentleness and resilience. Linked to mythology and nature through the river Aeron, it offers depth and earthy charm.

- **Aura:** With Latin and Greek roots, Aura means "gentle breeze" or "wind," embodying tranquility and clarity. Connected to the Greek goddess of breezes, this name offers an ethereal and serene presence.

- **Autumn:** A Latin-origin name meaning "season of harvest," Autumn symbolizes reflection, transformation, and abundance. With its connection to nature's cycles and golden tones, it celebrates life's richness and beauty.

- **Blaze:** This bold, gender-neutral name of Latin origin means "fire" or "flame." Blaze embodies passion and individuality, offering a modern and dynamic choice for parents seeking fiery energy.

- **Clay:** An earthy name of Old English origin, Clay represents strength and malleability. Its connection to the earth gives it a grounded and enduring appeal. With its short, solid sound, Clay feels both modern and timeless.

- **Cove:** A gender-neutral name of British origin, Cove means "small coastal inlet" and connects to the tranquility of sheltered bays. With serene and adventurous imagery, this evocative name carries peace and courage.

- **Ember:** Of British origin, Ember means "spark" or "burning low," symbolizing warmth and quiet intensity. This gentle yet powerful name captures resilience and the enduring glow of a fire's remains.

- **Flora:** Of Latin origin, Flora means "flower" and honors the Roman goddess of spring and flowers. It symbolizes renewal, beauty, and growth, offering a vibrant, life-affirming name steeped in natural vitality.

- **Forrest:** Derived from the Old French forest ("woods"), Forrest embodies growth and resilience. It evokes imagery of strength, natural beauty, and adventure. This grounded, nature-inspired name has a timeless, rugged appeal.

- **Gaia:** Of Greek origin, Gaia is the personification of Earth and the mother of all life in mythology. It embodies growth, life, and nurturing, offering timeless strength and wisdom tied to the natural world.

- **Hazel:** Derived from the hazel tree, this Old English name carries warmth and heritage. Symbolizing wisdom and protection, Hazel offers a grounded and timeless connection to nature and Celtic traditions.

- **Lamar:** A name of French origin, meaning "the sea" or "dweller near water," Lamar carries a smooth, modern sound and evokes calm strength. Its unique tone and cultural significance add to its appeal.

- **Maris:** With Latin roots, meaning "of the sea," Maris evokes the calm mystery of the ocean. Linked to Stella Maris, "star of the sea," this poetic name honors grace and serenity, offering a connection to the sea's boundless energy.

- **Phoenix:** Of Greek origin, meaning "reborn," Phoenix symbolizes transformation and renewal. Associated with the mythological bird rising from ashes, it inspires strength and perseverance.

- **Rain:** A gentle, nature-inspired name of Old English and German origin, Rain symbolizes "abundance from above." Gender-neutral and serene, it evokes renewal, growth, and nurturing qualities, with variations like Raina, Rayne, and Reign adding versatility.

- **River:** Of English origin, meaning "a flowing body of water," River symbolizes life's journey, resilience, and adaptability. This tranquil, gender-neutral name reflects nature's strength and the peaceful beauty of flowing water, inspiring calmness and introspection.

- **Winter:** Of British and German origin, Winter symbolizes the magical season and is associated with stillness and transformation. Inspired by the "time of water," it captures purity and strength, making it a unique, nature-inspired choice.

- **Zephyr:** A gender-neutral name of Greek origin, meaning "west wind," Zephyr represents calm, freedom, and renewal. Tied to the gentle Greek god of the west wind, it evokes peace and natural grace.

- **Zinnia:** Named after the vibrant flower, Zinnia has German origins and symbolizes endurance, affection, and joy. Its bold, multi-colored bloom thrives in tough conditions, making it a lively and spirited choice for parents who value strength and beauty.

Names tied to the elements are more than just beautiful; they embody qualities that parents may hope will guide their child through life. These names inspire a sense of harmony, resilience, and purpose, mirroring the elements' dynamic roles in the world around us.

Mythological Names With Powerful Meanings

Mythological names hold a timeless appeal for parents who want their child's name to carry a sense of history, mystery, and strength. These names are steeped in stories of gods, goddesses, and legendary heroes whose virtues and achievements have inspired cultures for centuries. By choosing a mythological name, parents connect their children to the enduring themes of courage, wisdom, beauty, and resilience, qualities celebrated in myths and legends across the world. These names carry the power of ancient tales, embodying values and aspirations that give them both a sense of purpose and gravitas.

Here are some mythological names with rich meanings:

- **Aiden:** With Irish and Gaelic roots, Aiden means "little fire." Linked to the Celtic god of fire, Aodh, it represents warmth, energy, and vitality, offering a lively and spirited name with a timeless appeal.

- **Apollo:** Apollo, a name of Greek origin, honors the god of music, poetry, and healing. Associated with light and truth, Apollo embodies creativity and resilience, making it an ideal choice for parents drawn to artistry and a vibrant presence.

- **Artemis:** A Greek-origin name meaning "twin of Apollo," referring to the goddess of the moon, hunting, and wilderness, Artemis embodies strength, independence, and harmony with nature, inspiring resilience and adventure.

- **Athena:** Of Greek origin, Athena is named after the goddess of wisdom, war, and courage. As the patron goddess of Athens, she represents intelligence, strategy, and protection, blending strength and intellect for a name that inspires bravery and wisdom.

- **Aurora:** Meaning "dawn" in Latin, Aurora honors the Roman goddess of sunrise and the natural wonder of the aurora borealis. This radiant name symbolizes new beginnings, light, and a spirit of adventure.

- **Caelus:** This is a masculine name of Latin origin, meaning "sky" or "heavens." Rooted in Roman mythology, Caelus personified the celestial realm, connecting the name to the vastness and beauty of the stars.

- **Calista:** A name of Latin and Greek origin, meaning "most beautiful," Calista is tied to mythology and celestial imagery through the nymph Kallisto. Symbolizing grace and elegance, Calista celebrates beauty, both inner and outer.

- **Calliope:** A Greek name meaning "beautiful voice," Calliope honors the muse of epic poetry and creativity. Known for her eloquence and inspiration, this lyrical name exudes artistic charm and classical heritage.

- **Chloe:** From Greek origins, meaning "young green shoot" or "blooming," Chloe is associated with Demeter, the goddess of agriculture. It evokes springtime vitality and fertility, symbolizing growth and potential.

- **Damon:** Of Greek origin, Damon means "to tame" or "subdue." It is tied to the myth of Damon and Pythias, symbolizing loyalty and friendship. Damon's sleek, modern feel makes it a name of quiet strength and individuality.

- **Daphne:** From the Greek word for "laurel," Daphne is tied to mythological elegance. Its connection to nature and ancient stories gives it a unique allure. Rare and graceful, Daphne has a timeless sophistication.

- **Eirene:** Of Greek origin, meaning "peace," this name is tied to the goddess Eirene, who symbolized harmony and renewal. It inspires calm and balance, reflecting the goddess's tranquil spirit.

- **Elara:** Of Greek origin, Elara blends mythology and astronomy. A mortal princess in Greek lore and the name of one of Jupiter's moons, Elara symbolizes a connection between Earth and the cosmos.

- **Evander:** Meaning "good man" or "strong man" in Greek, Evander honors a Trojan war hero known for his strength and moral integrity. The name reflects both goodness and courage, making it an inspiring choice for parents seeking a virtuous name.

- **Freya:** A Norse name meaning "noble lady," Freya is the goddess of love, beauty, and fertility. Known for her bravery and compassion, Freya symbolizes strength and femininity, offering a name that balances grace and resilience.

- **Ikaros:** Ikaros is a Greek name meaning "the one who reaches the sky," inspired by the myth of Icarus, who flew too close to the sun. It represents ambition tempered by wisdom, making it a meaningful and mythologically rich choice.

- **Juno:** Of Latin origin, Juno means "queen of the gods" and "youthful." A Roman goddess who protected women and marriage, Juno embodies strength, loyalty, and tradition, making it a great choice for parents valuing family and grace.

- **Leander:** Of Greek origin, Leander means "lion-man," symbolizing courage and loyalty. Inspired by the myth of Leander, who braved the seas for love, this heroic name offers a unique alternative to classics like Alexander.

- **Loki:** A Norse name meaning "lock," this name is associated with the god of mischief. Known for his cunning and transformative abilities, Loki represents adaptability and the power of reinvention, offering an edgy and modern mythological appeal.

- **Luna:** Of Latin origin, meaning "moon," Luna is inspired by the Roman goddess who drove her chariot across the sky. Symbolizing independence and radiance, Luna carries timeless celestial charm.

- **Lyra:** A Greek name meaning "lyre," Lyra is tied to the constellation and the myth of Orpheus, whose music enchanted gods and nature. This celestial and musical name inspires creativity and poetic allure.

- **Maeve:** Of Irish origin, meaning "intoxicating" or "she who rules," Maeve is rooted in mythology as the powerful Queen of Connacht.

This name conveys beauty, strength, and ambition, enriched by its connection to Irish folklore.

- **Odin:** Of Old Norse origin, Odin is the all-father god in Norse mythology, associated with wisdom, war, and magic. The name reflects strength, relentless pursuit of knowledge, and a connection to mystical realms, embodying divine inspiration and courage.

- **Orion:** Named after the great hunter in Greek mythology, Orion is also a celestial constellation symbolizing adventure and curiosity. This name evokes the majesty of the night sky and a spirit of exploration, ideal for parents inspired by celestial beauty.

- **Selene:** This Greek name means "the moon" and honors the goddess who illuminated the night sky with her chariot. Selene embodies tranquility, beauty, and the mystery of moonlight.

- **Thora:** Of Scandinavian origin, Thora means "thunder" and is linked to the Norse god Thor, protector of humanity and god of thunder. Bold and graceful, Thora is a mythological name that embodies strength and resilience.

- **Vesta:** A Latin name associated with the Roman goddess of the hearth, Vesta means "to abide" and reflects nurturing and protective qualities. Revered in Roman culture, it symbolizes warmth, family, and tradition.

These mythological names offer not just beauty but also profound meanings rooted in ancient stories that have shaped human history. Names like Athena and Apollo celebrate creativity and courage, while Freya and Odin embody strength and wisdom. Each of these names provides a sense of connection to enduring ideals and legends, giving a child a name that is both inspiring and timeless.

Wrapping Up

Nature-inspired and mythological names provide a meaningful connection to the beauty of the natural world and the timeless stories of mythology. These names carry an essence of grounding, resilience, and mystery, linking children to qualities celebrated in nature and ancient lore. You can give your child a name with layers of significance, offering both strength and inspiration drawn from the earth and history's legendary figures by choosing a nature-inspired or mythological name.

While we touched on a few gender-neutral and modern names, the next chapter takes a deeper look into them. Join us as we explore contemporary and versatile options that reflect today's values of inclusivity, individuality, and adaptability, offering names that blend tradition with a fresh perspective!

Chapter 5:
Modern and Gender-Neutral Names

As naming traditions evolve, modern and gender-neutral names have emerged as a reflection of today's values. These names challenge traditional conventions, celebrating inclusivity, individuality, and adaptability. For parents, choosing a modern or gender-neutral name isn't just about breaking boundaries—it's about giving their child the freedom to grow into their identity, unconfined by societal expectations.

Unlike classic or nature-inspired names explored in earlier chapters, modern and gender-neutral options combine creativity with versatility. Names like Rowan, Avery, and Zion offer adaptability across contexts, while others such as Harper, Reese, and Kai resonate with contemporary ideals of inclusivity. These names reflect a fresh, innovative spirit while maintaining a timeless appeal.

Modern and gender-neutral names empower children by transcending stereotypes, encouraging them to define themselves on their own terms. Choosing such a name ensures your child will carry an identity as dynamic and unique as they are—a name that resonates today and remains relevant in the future.

The Growing Popularity of Gender-Neutral Names

Baby names are undergoing a revolution. If you've met a child named Blake or Jordan and wondered about their gender, you've already seen the rise of gender-neutral naming. These names reflect a broader societal shift toward individuality and inclusivity, making them a powerful statement in today's world.

This trend stems from parents increasingly seeking unique, modern names. Over the past century, naming conventions have moved away from traditional patterns. For instance, in the 1880s, nearly a third of all babies were given one of the top ten names of the time. By 2020, that figure dropped to just seven percent (Zhang, 2023). The rise of gender-neutral names reflects a shift in how society views identity. These names celebrate versatility and individuality, marking a moment in naming trends where inclusivity takes center stage.

Here are some popular gender-neutral examples:

- **Avery:** A British-origin name meaning "elf counsel" or "ruler of elves," Avery carries a whimsical and magical connotation. Its sleek, modern sound across cultures makes it a popular choice for parents seeking a gender-neutral name.

- **Casey:** Of Irish origin, Casey means "vigilant" or "watchful." Historically a surname, Casey is a versatile, gender-neutral name associated with resilience and attentiveness.

- **Emerson:** Meaning "son of Emery," Emerson is of German origin. This name is linked to the literary legacy of poet Ralph Waldo Emerson, embodying intellectual depth and creative spirit.

- **Emery:** Derived from the Germanic name Emmerich, Emery means "industrious leader." It's widely embraced as a gender-neutral name with a subtle nature-inspired vibe. Its modern charm and adaptability ensure lasting popularity.

- **Finley:** Of Scottish and Irish origin, Finley means "fair warrior." Traditionally a Celtic surname, it has evolved into a charming first name, reflecting both bravery and gentleness.

- **Harlow:** A name of Old English origin, Harlow means "army hill." With its edgy yet elegant vibe, it's a gender-neutral choice that conveys strength and sophistication.

- **Jordan:** A biblical name of Hebrew origin, Jordan means "to flow down" or "descending" and is tied to the River Jordan, a significant site in Christianity. Its spiritual nature gives it a deep historical resonance, making it an enduring choice for families valuing strength, faith, and inclusivity.

- **Kendall:** Of Old English origin, meaning "valley of the River Kent," Kendall is sleek and modern. Its stylish tone makes it an excellent gender-neutral name with historical roots. Kendall's adaptability ensures its enduring charm.

- **Raelyn:** A modern combination of "Rae" and "Lyn," this name conveys softness and individuality. Raelyn is a versatile choice that blends contemporary style with gender-neutral appeal.

- **Riley:** With British and Irish origins, Riley means "rye clearing" or "courageous." Its connection to strength and heritage, derived from the Irish surname Reilly, adds depth and meaning. This empowering name is bold, versatile, and appealing to children of any gender.

- **Rowan:** With Irish and Scottish roots, Rowan means "little redhead" and connects to the rowan tree, which symbolizes protection and enchantment in folklore. This versatile name suits fiery personalities and has a nature-inspired charm that balances strength and elegance.

- **Sawyer:** Meaning "woodcutter," Sawyer is of English origin. Originally an occupational surname, it has evolved into a gender-neutral name with an adventurous, grounded feel.

- **Saylor:** Meaning "sailor" or "boatman," this occupational name of English origin conveys a spirit of adventure and freedom. It's a fresh, gender-neutral choice with nautical charm.

- **Scout:** A gender-neutral name of Old French origin, meaning "to listen," Scout embodies curiosity and exploration. Popularized by *To Kill a Mockingbird,* it reflects intelligence and adventurous spirit.

- **Skyler:** Derived from the Dutch surname Schuyler, meaning "scholar," Skyler is a gender-neutral name with intellectual and airy qualities, reflecting curiosity and creativity. Variants include "Skylar", which makes it an ideal name for parents seeking elegance, versatility, and educational inspiration.

- **Sutton***:* Sutton is an Old English name that means "from the southern homestead." Once a place name, it has transitioned into a sleek first name, symbolizing roots and refinement.

- **Taylor:** Of French origin, Taylor means "tailor" or "to cut." It started as an occupational surname but has evolved into a stylish given name. Taylor's association with craftsmanship and creativity, coupled with its modern appeal from figures like Taylor Swift and Taylor Lautner, ensures its gender-neutral charm.

- **Teagan:** Of Irish origin, Teagan means "little poet" or "beautiful." Its lyrical sound and rich heritage make it a gender-neutral name that balances tradition and modernity.

- **Wren:** Inspired by the small, songbird, Wren is an Old English name symbolizing freedom and

95

creativity. Its simplicity and connection to nature make it a timeless, gender-neutral option.

Gender-neutral names like these offer a harmonious blend of history, meaning, and adaptability. They reflect the values of a world that increasingly celebrates individuality and inclusivity, giving children a name that empowers them to embrace their unique identity.

Flexibility and Inclusivity of Gender-Neutral Names

Gender-neutral names offer flexibility, adapting effortlessly to a child's evolving identity and life path. They allow children to express themselves authentically, whether embracing traditional roles or challenging societal norms. Names like Harper, Finn, and Parker transcend gender boundaries with ease, fitting various stages of life and contexts.

Consider names like:

- **Addison:** Originally an English surname meaning "son of Adam," Addison has evolved into a stylish unisex name. Its modern feel and soft yet strong sound contribute to its widespread appeal. Addison combines tradition with contemporary versatility.

- **Arden:** An Old English name meaning "valley of the eagle," Arden carries natural sophistication. Its minimalist sound gives it a modern, gender-neutral edge. Arden is ideal for those seeking a name that blends nature and style.

- **Baylor:** Of Old English origin, Baylor means "deliverer of goods." Known for its practicality, Baylor symbolizes dependability and ingenuity, offering a forward-thinking and gender-neutral choice.

- **Fallon:** Of Irish origin, Fallon means "leader" or "descendant of Fallamhan." This gender-neutral name reflects strength and charisma with a fresh, contemporary vibe.

- **Finn:** Rooted in Irish mythology, Finn means "fair" or "blessed" and is tied to the legendary warrior Fionn, who symbolizes wisdom and courage. Its concise and multicultural ties, with Scandinavian meaning "from Finland," give Finn a timeless charm that fits any gender.

- **Gray:** A sleek, minimalist name of English origin, Gray refers to the color and symbolizes neutrality, balance, and calm. Its modern, gender-neutral appeal makes it a stylish choice.

- **Harper:** A British-origin name meaning "harpist" or "minstrel," Harper connects to the artistry of medieval entertainers and musicians. Its harmonious essence and creative flair make it a favorite for families who cherish music and the arts.

- **Hayden:** An Old English name meaning "heather-covered hill," Hayden has natural elegance. Its soft yet strong sound gives it a modern, gender-neutral charm. Hayden's versatility makes it a popular choice for contemporary parents.

- **Kiran:** Of Sanskrit origin, meaning "ray of light," Kiran exudes positivity and elegance. Its cultural depth and universal sound make it a rare and versatile option. Kiran's simplicity and brightness ensure its lasting appeal.

- **Landry:** Landry is a French name meaning "ruler" or "landowner." Grounded in historical roots, it carries connotations of leadership and versatility, with a modern touch that resonates across genders.

- **Leighton:** Of Old English origin, Leighton means "meadow town." This name merges pastoral imagery with a modern edge, reflecting a harmonious balance of tradition and contemporary style.

- **Leslie:** A Scottish name meaning "garden of holly," this nature-inspired name carries a serene charm and historical significance, having been embraced across generations as a unisex option.

- **Logan:** A Scottish name meaning "hollow," Logan has grown beyond its geographic origins to symbolize strength, independence, and resilience. With ties to pop culture, including the iconic film *Logan*, the name carries a futuristic, heroic appeal while maintaining a versatile and approachable quality.

- **Luca:** An Italian and Latin name meaning "bringer of light," Luca is warm and inviting. Its international appeal and modern tone give it a unique, unisex versatility. Luca is both stylish and timeless, making it a beloved choice.

- **Maren:** A Latin and Scandinavian name meaning "sea," Maren embodies the calm and power of the ocean, making it a great choice with a connection to nature and inner peace.

- **Morgan:** Of Welsh origin, Morgan means "circling sea" or "white sea dweller." Rooted in Celtic mythology, where it's associated with the Morrígan, a goddess of war and fate, Morgan carries strength, determination, and rich cultural significance, making it a lasting and flexible choice.

- **Nico:** Derived from the Italian form of the Greek name Nicholas, Nico means "victory of the people." Its sleek simplicity and association with strength and triumph make it a standout gender-neutral name. Nico's versatility ensures it works well across cultures and as a diminutive or standalone name.

- **Parker:** Of British origin, Parker means "park keeper" and evokes connections to nature, freedom, and playfulness. Originally an occupational surname, Parker has transitioned into a modern, balanced name that is suitable for children of any gender.

- **Peyton:** Derived from Old English, Peyton means "fighting man's estate." A versatile name, it conveys resilience and poise, widely adopted for its balance of tradition and contemporary style.

- **Presley:** Of English origin, Presley means "priest's meadow." It carries a vibrant cultural significance due to its association with Elvis Presley, blending musical legacy with modern sensibility.

- **Rory:** Of Irish origin, Rory means "red king." Traditionally a male name, it has become a dynamic, gender-neutral choice associated with vitality and creativity, notably connected to Rory Gilmore from *Gilmore Girls*.

- **Ryan:** Of Irish origin, meaning "little king," Ryan is a classic yet modern unisex name. Its straightforward sound and strong roots contribute to its timeless appeal. Ryan's adaptability ensures its continued relevance across generations.

- **Tatum:** Of Old English origin, Tatum means "cheerful bringer of joy." This playful, gender-neutral name combines elegance and warmth, making it a versatile choice.

The inclusivity of gender-neutral names lies in their ability to bridge tradition and innovation. For families, these names represent a commitment to raising children in a world that values diversity and freedom of expression.

Modern Names Reflecting Current Trends

Modern baby names often reflect the cultural and technological shifts of the present. Names like Nova, Hunter, and Quinn resonate with contemporary values and ideals. They are versatile, gender-neutral, and globally appealing.

Here are names that transcend traditional boundaries:

- **Alexis:** Of Greek origin, meaning "defender," Alexis is a bold yet elegant name. Its widespread use across genders adds to its modern versatility. With its strong roots and approachable tone, Alexis remains a popular choice.

- **Braxton:** Braxton is an English-origin name meaning "Brock's town." With its bold sound and modern flair, this name has become a popular choice, blending tradition with a confident, contemporary vibe.

- **Carter:** Meaning "transporter of goods by cart," this British-origin name blends practicality and sophistication. Recognized through figures like U.S. President Jimmy Carter, it carries associations of hard work and creativity, with a touch of luxury through connections to Cartier.

- **Crew:** An English word name, Crew symbolizes teamwork and camaraderie. Its modern, straightforward vibe makes it a rising favorite for parents seeking a fresh, strong choice.

- **Easton:** Of English origin, meaning "east-facing town," Easton exudes charm and strength. Its stylish sound makes it a top pick for parents looking for modern yet traditional balance.

- **Hendrix:** Inspired by the legendary musician Jimi Hendrix, this Dutch-origin name meaning "son of Hendrick" conveys creativity and boldness with a rock-and-roll edge.

- **Hudson:** An English name meaning "son of Hugh," Hudson is a strong, nature-inspired name linked to the famous river. Its timeless appeal and modern edge make it a favorite.

- **Hunter:** A British-origin name meaning "one who hunts," Hunter reflects strength, independence, and a connection to nature. Originally an occupational surname, it now appeals as a bold, gender-neutral choice embodying self-sufficiency and resourcefulness with a contemporary edge.

- **Jett:** Jett is of English origin, meaning "black mineral." With its sleek, high-energy vibe, this name is a bold choice, perfect for parents seeking a name with modern charisma and strength.

- **Jude:** Of Hebrew origin, Jude means "praised." A short and timeless name with biblical roots, it is associated with strength and loyalty. Known for its cultural appeal, Jude resonates as a modern, gender-neutral option that balances simplicity and depth.

- **Knox:** Knox is a Scottish-origin name meaning "round hill." Rugged and strong, it gained prominence through its celebrity connections and is celebrated for its concise yet commanding sound.

- **Landon:** An Old English name meaning "long hill," Landon blends nature with modernity. Its strong yet approachable sound makes it a popular gender-neutral choice. Landon exudes a contemporary and adventurous energy.

- **Lennon:** Of Irish origin, Lennon means "lover" or "descendant of Leannán." Closely tied to music legend John Lennon, it reflects creativity, individuality, and a message of peace and love.

- **Maddox:** Of Welsh origin, Maddox means "son of Madoc" or "fortunate." With its edgy, adventurous tone, Maddox is a name that stands out, symbolizing boldness and luck with a touch of sophistication.

- **Milo:** With Germanic roots meaning "merciful" or "soldier," Milo is a soft yet strong name. Its growing popularity reflects its charm as a gender-neutral name that conveys kindness and bravery.

- **Nova:** Of Latin origin, meaning "new," Nova symbolizes new beginnings and limitless potential. Its celestial ties to sudden, bright stars add wonder and innovation, making it a modern yet timeless choice for a child representing a fresh chapter in life.

- **Paxton:** An Old English name meaning "peaceful town" and known for its soothing yet strong qualities, Paxton conveys a sense of harmony and strength, rooted in history but fitting for modern times.

- **Quinn:** Of Gaelic origin, meaning "chief," "counsel," or "wisdom," Quinn is a sleek, gender-neutral name with rich heritage. Its contemporary feel and versatile sound make it a standout in both media and literature, symbolizing intelligence and leadership.

- **Reese:** Reese is a Welsh name meaning "enthusiasm," "fire," and "ardor." Its fiery connotation inspires ambition, making it a dynamic, gender-neutral option for parents seeking a name that reflects drive and vitality.

- **Zion:** This Hebrew name meaning "highest point" holds deep spiritual significance, symbolizing utopia and ultimate achievement. Associated with hope, resilience, and empowerment, Zion resonates as a name full of inspiration and ambition, with modern appeal through its use in pop culture and music.

Modern names like these capture the essence of what it means to live in today's world. They are inclusive and imbued with meanings that serve as reminders of innovation, strength, and individuality, ensuring they remain relevant and cherished for years to come.

The Appeal of Simplicity and Versatility in Modern and Gender-Neutral Names

Parents increasingly favor names that are simple, adaptable, and globally understood. These names bridge tradition and modernity, ensuring practicality and universal appeal. Names like Blake, Tate, and Kai exemplify how brevity can convey depth.

Each of these names is imbued with rich meanings and cultural significance, proving that brevity can carry profound resonance:

- **Archer:** Of English origin, Archer means "bowman." Evoking imagery of precision and strength, Archer combines historical roots with a sense of modern adventure and determination.

- **Arlo:** A name of Old English and Spanish origins, Arlo means "fortified hill" or "barberry tree." Its simplicity and connection to nature give it a grounded, gender-neutral charm.

- **Blake:** Of British origin, meaning "dark," "black," or "pale," Blake's dual meanings reflect balance and versatility. Known for its artistic ties, such as to poet William Blake, this modern and crisp name appeals for its intriguing depth and adaptability.

- **Callum:** A Scottish name meaning "dove," Callum symbolizes peace and gentleness. Its soft sound and rich heritage make it an enduringly appealing choice.

- **Camden:** Of Scottish origin, Camden means "winding valley." This modern, gender-neutral name has a stylish yet grounded appeal, perfect for those drawn to nature.

- **Chase:** Of Old French origin, meaning "to hunt," Chase exudes energy and action. Its sleek and modern feel makes it a versatile, unisex choice. With its dynamic tone, Chase conveys determination and individuality.

- **Dawsen:** A variant of Dawson, meaning "son of David," this updated version of a traditional name blends a sense of lineage with a contemporary edge, offering strength and individuality.

- **Gia:** Derived from Italian and Greek origins, Gia means "God is gracious." This compact and elegant name carries an international flair, balancing simplicity with timeless warmth and sophistication.

- **Kai:** A globally resonant name, Kai has meanings across cultures: "sea" in Hawaiian, "food" in Māori, and "nature or harmony" in Scandinavian and Japanese traditions. This name symbolizes vastness, beauty, and essential life connections.

- **Lin:** Primarily of Chinese origin, Lin means "forest" or "fine jade," symbolizing nature and preciousness. Its serene simplicity and cultural adaptability, with meanings like "brightness" in Burmese and ties to "linden hill" in English, make it a versatile choice.

- **Lincoln:** Lincoln is an old English name meaning "lake colony." Often associated with President Abraham Lincoln, it reflects leadership, historical gravitas, and enduring dignity, making it a powerful choice.

- **Max:** Derived from the Latin *Maximilianus*, meaning "greatest," Max is a versatile, approachable name. Its concise form carries power and charm, making it a popular, gender-neutral choice with a timeless quality.

- **Noelle:** A French name meaning "Christmas," Noelle reflects joy and celebration. It's a name with timeless elegance and warmth, perfect for the holiday season or beyond.

- **Ori:** A deeply inclusive name with Hebrew origins, meaning "my light," Ori embodies spiritual guidance. Its multicultural significance spans Japanese and Yoruba cultures, symbolizing destiny and intuition, making it a globally meaningful and versatile choice.

- **Tanner:** This is an English occupational name meaning "leatherworker." With its rugged and straightforward nature, Tanner evokes practicality and resilience while remaining stylish and approachable.

- **Tate:** Meaning "cheerful" in its British origins, Tate's simplicity and one-syllable form make it approachable and universally positive. Its history as a given name and nickname adds staying power, appealing to parents who value friendliness.

Modern and gender-neutral names are attractive because they embody a rare combination of simplicity and depth. They are short yet powerful, easy to use yet rich in meaning, and inherently versatile.

Empowering Children With Names That Defy Stereotypes

A child's name is their first introduction to the world, shaping both how they are perceived and how they perceive themselves. Gender-neutral names are particularly empowering, freeing children from societal constraints and opening doors to diverse opportunities. Research from Columbia Business School (CBS Newsroom, 2016) shows that names influence gender assumptions and treatment. Choosing gender-neutral names like Ellis or Sloan provides a clean slate, allowing children to explore interests, careers, and identities without predefined expectations.

These names also reduce bias in professional contexts, offering inclusivity, adaptability, and a sense of empowerment:

- **Cameron:** Of Scottish origin, meaning "crooked nose," Cameron's historical roots as a clan leader's name blend with modern versatility. Popular across cultures and professions, this name embodies strength, adaptability, and flexibility.

- **Dylan:** A Welsh name meaning "great tide" or "son of the sea," Dylan reflects adaptability and resilience. Linked to Welsh mythology and the sea god, it symbolizes exploration and strength, with growing appeal as a versatile, gender-neutral option.

- **Ellis:** Of Welsh, Greek, and Hebrew origin, Ellis means "kind" or "benevolent." With ties to the Hebrew name Eliyahu ("Jehovah is God") and American history through Ellis Island, this name is a meaningful choice for cultural integration and kindness.

- **Grant:** From Old French, meaning "great" or "tall," Grant is a name of quiet strength. Its short, impactful sound adds to its modern appeal and versatility. Grant is a timeless choice that balances simplicity with sophistication.

- **Hallie:** A modern variation of the Old English name Hayley, Hallie means "dweller in the hay meadow." Its soft and approachable sound gives it a friendly and unisex quality. Hallie blends vintage roots with contemporary style.

- **Hollis:** A British-origin name meaning "holly trees," Hollis evokes strength, beauty, and resilience. Associated with the vibrant holly tree, it symbolizes protection and endurance while offering a festive, timeless appeal connected to nature.

- **Jovie:** Inspired by "jovial," Jovie conveys cheerfulness and lightheartedness. This uplifting and modern gender-neutral name radiates positivity, making it perfect for a child full of joy and energy.

- **Keegan:** Keegan is an Irish name meaning "descendant of Aodhagán" or "fiery." With its energetic and vibrant tone, it blends Irish heritage with a spirited and versatile modern touch.

- **Nash:** Of English origin, Nash means "by the ash tree." This sleek, nature-inspired name combines simplicity with contemporary style, offering a grounded yet modern option.

- **Onyx:** A name of Greek origin, Onyx refers to the precious black gemstone. It symbolizes strength and resilience, offering a bold and modern gender-neutral choice.

- **Paisley:** A Scottish name referring to the distinctive textile pattern and symbolizing creativity and artistic flair, Paisley offers a charming and whimsical choice rooted in cultural history.

- **Remington:** Of Old English origin, Remington means "place on a riverbank." Originally a surname, this bold, gender-neutral name has a modern and sophisticated appeal, symbolizing resilience and adventure.

- **Rhett:** Of Dutch origin, Rhett means "advice" or "counsel." Evoking strength and sophistication, Rhett carries literary significance from *Gone with the Wind*, adding depth to its bold and classic nature.

- **Sasha:** Of Russian origin, Sasha is a diminutive of Alexander or Alexandra, meaning "defender of men." This gender-neutral name is chic and cosmopolitan, with a soft yet bold presence. Its global appeal and versatility make it both rare and accessible.

- **Silas:** Derived from Latin and Greek origins, Silas means "forest" or "wood." This name carries a rustic charm and a connection to nature, exuding strength and resilience.

- **Sloan:** Derived from Irish origins, Sloan means "raider" or "warrior." Rich in heritage, it symbolizes bravery, resilience, and leadership, offering a gender-neutral name that connects to ancient Irish traditions and inspires strength and courage.

Choosing a name like Hollis, Dylan, or Cameron allows parents to challenge traditional notions of gender and provide their child with an identity unbound by stereotypes. These names encourage confidence and flexibility, enabling children to define their own paths in life.

Wrapping Up

Modern and gender-neutral names represent a cultural shift towards inclusivity, individuality, and freedom of identity. These names challenge societal norms, offering children the flexibility to grow into unique individuals unbound by traditional expectations. They adapt seamlessly across cultures, ages, and contexts, ensuring that children are equipped with names that grow alongside them.

However, while modern names push boundaries and challenge conventions, many parents also find profound inspiration in the time-honored traditions and deep meanings of spiritual, biblical, and cultural names. In the next chapter, we'll explore the enduring appeal of these meaningful names and the stories they carry.

Chapter 6:
Spiritual, Biblical, and Cultural Names

When choosing a name for their child, many parents look for options that reflect their beliefs, heritage, or traditions. Spiritual, biblical, and cultural names offer that connection. Rich in history and meaning, these names embody timeless values, family traditions, and a sense of belonging to a larger community.

In this chapter, you'll discover names with profound significance, linking your child to faith, virtue, and identity. Biblical names like Elijah or Grace serve as daily reminders of divine blessings, while cultural names like Santiago or Amina honor heritage and celebrate the traditions that shape us. These names tell stories, connecting children to their roots while offering a sense of purpose and belonging.

Whether you're drawn to a name from scripture, a virtue name, or one that celebrates your cultural legacy, this chapter will guide you toward finding a meaningful choice that resonates with your family's journey.

The Deep Meaning Behind Spiritual and Biblical Names

For many parents, spiritual and biblical names reflect faith and timeless values. Often drawn from sacred texts, these names symbolize virtues like strength, grace, and wisdom—qualities parents hope their children will embody. Names like Noah or Faith are daily reminders of kindness, perseverance, and spiritual strength, while Eve connects to enduring lessons of courage and resilience.

Spiritual and biblical names often bridge the past, present, and future. Passed down through centuries, they represent unchanging values in an ever-changing world. These names also foster a sense of identity, serving as beacons during challenges and reminders of the values instilled by family. Choosing a spiritual or biblical name connects your child to their roots while inspiring them to live a life of purpose.

Here are a few names with profound spiritual significance:

- **Abel:** A Hebrew name meaning "breath" or "vapor," Abel is a timeless biblical name symbolizing humility and the fleeting yet precious nature of life, offering spiritual depth and simplicity.

- **Angelo:** An Italian name meaning "angel" or "messenger," Angelo exudes spiritual significance. Its melodic sound reflects divine connection and grace. Angelo carries an elegant yet approachable charm that is enriched by its cultural ties.

- **Ariel:** Of Hebrew origin, Ariel means "lion of God." Biblically associated with Jerusalem and symbolic of strength and protection, its graceful tone and spiritual depth make it a timeless, versatile choice.

- **Asher:** Of Hebrew origin, Asher means "blessed" and "happy." As a biblical name, it highlights prosperity and joy, while its Old English ties to the ash tree symbolize strength and growth. Asher blends faith with nature's resilience.

- **Bodhi:** Of Sanskrit origin, Bodhi means "awakening" or "enlightenment." Deeply tied to Buddhist philosophy, it symbolizes spiritual growth and mindfulness. Its serene and meaningful tone makes it a modern, unique choice.

- **Camila:** Meaning "religious attendant" or "priest's helper," Camila is of Latin origin and tied to devotion and service. Its historical connections to ancient Rome add depth, while diminutives like Milla and Millie bring warmth and timeless elegance.

- **Charity:** This British virtue name means "giving" or "kindness." Popular during the Puritan era, it emphasizes selflessness and compassion, making it a meaningful and unique choice for instilling generosity.

- **Delilah:** This name is of Hebrew origin, meaning "delicate." Known for its soft, lyrical quality, Delilah carries a blend of elegance and historical intrigue, tied to its rich biblical narrative.

- **Eden:** Derived from Hebrew, meaning "delight" or "paradise," Eden is closely associated with the biblical Garden of Eden, representing natural beauty, beginnings, and innocence.

- **Eliana:** A name of Hebrew and Latin origins, Eliana means "God has answered" and reflects gratitude and divine inspiration. In Latin, it connects to "sun," evoking vitality and celestial energy. Eliana combines spirituality with natural imagery, offering luminous strength and versatility.

- **Eve:** Meaning "life" or "living being," Eve originates from Hebrew and Latin roots. It celebrates creation and vitality, tied to the biblical story of the first woman. Eve is a simple yet profound name honoring beginnings and humanity's strength.

- **Ezra:** A Hebrew name meaning "Yah helps" or "help," Ezra honors the biblical scribe who restored the Jewish community after exile. This name reflects perseverance and spiritual depth, offering a humble yet profound choice for parents.

- **Faith:** This English name, meaning "trust" or "devotion," has been cherished as a virtue name since the 17th century. Reflecting loyalty and steadfast values, Faith inspires strength and spiritual commitment.

- **Gabriel:** Of Hebrew origin, meaning "man of God," Gabriel is steeped in spiritual significance as the name of the Archangel Gabriel in Christianity and Islam. Known for delivering divine messages, Gabriel symbolizes faith and creativity. Nicknames like Gabe add a gentle, modern touch to its rich legacy.

- **Hannah:** A Hebrew name meaning "grace" or "favor," Hannah is a cherished biblical name that represents kindness, faith, and spiritual blessings, resonating with enduring strength and warmth.

- **Harmony:** Of Greek origin, meaning "agreement" or "unity," Harmony represents balance, peace, and a musical connection to life's rhythms, making it a name that resonates with serenity.

- **Hope:** This British virtue name means "confidence" or "trust." Popularized by Puritans, it signifies resilience and optimism. Hope inspires a fresh perspective, encouraging positivity and grace in embracing life's possibilities.

- **Jasper:** Derived from Persian, meaning "treasurer," Jasper is tied to one of the Three Wise Men. Its connection to gemstones symbolizes beauty and value. Jasper's sleek, modern tone ensures it remains timeless and appealing.

- **Joaquim:** Of Hebrew origin, meaning "God has established," Joaquim is a strong and spiritual name. Its Portuguese and Spanish roots give it a unique, international flair. Joaquim's regal and refined tone makes it a distinctive choice.

- **Jubilee:** A name of Hebrew origin, meaning "celebration" or "rejoicing," Jubilee symbolizes freedom and renewal. Its vibrant energy makes it a name filled with positivity and joy, perfect for a child who inspires happiness.

- **Leah:** A timeless Hebrew name meaning "weary" or "delicate," Leah is a biblical name that signifies devotion and perseverance. It is beloved for its simplicity and enduring elegance.

- **Levi:** A Hebrew name meaning "joined," Levi is tied to biblical history as the third son of Jacob and Leah. Balancing tradition with modernity, it is both a spiritual and stylish choice.

- **Matthew:** Meaning "gift of God," this Hebrew name is tied to Saint Matthew, an apostle and gospel author. Rooted in faith and gratitude,

Matthew combines classic charm with modern adaptability, including variations like Matteo.

- **Michael:** A Hebrew name meaning "who resembles God?" Michael is steeped in religious significance, representing protection and strength as the name of the archangel leading heaven's armies. Universally revered, it is a powerful and enduring choice.

- **Moses:** Of Hebrew origin, meaning "drawn out," Moses is tied to the iconic biblical leader. It symbolizes faith, strength, and deliverance. Moses's spiritual significance and classic tone make it a powerful choice.

- **Nathaniel:** Of Hebrew origin, Nathaniel means "God has given." With mentions in both the Old and New Testament, it symbolizes faith and gratitude. Timeless yet modern, it is often shortened to Nate for a contemporary appeal.

- **Noah:** A Hebrew name with dual meanings of "rest" and "motion," Noah honors the biblical figure known for resilience and faith while also reflecting vitality and balance. It is a timeless name symbolizing harmony between stillness and progress.

- **Rafael:** A Hebrew name meaning "God has healed," Rafael is tied to the archangel in biblical tradition. Its spiritual significance reflects healing and divine protection. With variations like Raphael and Raffaele, it carries global appeal and timeless elegance.

- **Ruth:** Meaning "friend," Ruth is a Hebrew name symbolizing love, kindness, and faithfulness. A significant biblical figure as King David's great-grandmother, Ruth exemplifies loyalty and compassion. Its enduring qualities make it a cherished name across generations and cultures.

- **Selah:** Of Hebrew origin, meaning "pause" or "reflection," Selah appears in the Psalms as a poetic term inviting contemplation. It embodies peace and spiritual stillness, making it a thoughtful and meaningful choice.

- **Seraphim:** A Hebrew name meaning "the burning one," Seraphim symbolizes divine strength and love. Associated with the highest-ranking angels in Judaism, Christianity, and Islam, it reflects intense devotion and spiritual passion, inspiring a life of faith and purpose.

- **Serenity:** A virtue name of French and Latin origin, Serenity means "peaceful" or "calm." It reflects grace, balance, and inner strength, encouraging a tranquil life of resilience and clarity.

- **Shiloh:** A Hebrew name meaning "tranquil" and "His gift," Shiloh carries deep biblical significance as a place of peace and divine assembly. Known as the dwelling of the Ark of the Covenant, it symbolizes serenity and spiritual abundance.

- **Tabitha:** Tabitha is an Aramaic name meaning "gazelle." Reflecting both elegance and agility, it is rooted in biblical compassion and grace, embodying a sense of beauty and resilience.

- **Talia:** A name of Hebrew origin, meaning "dew from heaven," Talia carries a gentle, spiritual significance. It is also linked to Greek roots, where it means "blooming" or "flourishing." Talia's soft, melodic sound and cultural depth make it a cherished name.

- **Zachary:** Derived from Hebrew Zechariah, meaning "the Lord recalled," Zachary blends biblical roots with contemporary charm. Its friendly nicknames Zach, Zack, and Zak enhance its modern appeal, while its strong heritage ensures lasting significance.

Choosing a spiritual or biblical name is a meaningful way to connect your child to a legacy of faith, values, and timeless virtues. These names are rich in history and significance, reflecting parents' deep-seated aspirations for their children: to live lives marked by grace and moral strength.

How Names Connect to Historical and Religious Figures

Spiritual and biblical names are often linked to influential figures, offering a connection to admired legacies. Names like Abraham or Mohammed resonate with the strong character and achievements of historical and religious figures. They carry values like resilience, wisdom, and compassion that have shaped societies and inspired generations.

Choosing such a name grounds a child in stories of strength and purpose. For instance:

- **Abraham:** A Hebrew name meaning "high father" or "father of multitudes," Abraham reflects leadership and faith, honoring the biblical patriarch and historical figures like Abraham Lincoln.

- **Aisha:** An Arabic name meaning "alive and well," Aisha reflects vitality and is cherished for its connection to the prophet Muhammad's wife. Its versatility makes it a meaningful choice.

- **Audrey:** Of Old English origin, Audrey means "noble strength." Famous through figures like Saint Audrey and Audrey Hepburn, it combines grace and resilience. Its vintage charm and modern relevance make it a timeless favorite.

- **Brigid:** Of Irish origin, meaning "strength" or "exalted one," Brigid is tied to Celtic mythology as a goddess of poetry, healing, and fire, symbolizing creativity and resilience.

- **Caleb:** Of Hebrew origin, Caleb means "wholehearted" or "faithful." It is tied to the biblical figure who displayed loyalty and courage as a companion of Moses. Caleb's timeless simplicity and spiritual depth ensure its lasting appeal.

- **Casimir:** Of Slavic origin, meaning "proclaimer of peace," Casimir combines strength and diplomacy. It carries royal associations, offering a regal and distinguished flair.

- **Christopher:** Of Greek origin, meaning "bearing Christ," this name holds deep spiritual significance and honors Saint Christopher, the protector of travelers. Timeless and versatile, it symbolizes guidance and strength.

- **Dante:** Derived from the Latin word for "steadfast," Dante represents resilience and creativity and is associated with Dante Alighieri and his literary masterpiece, *The Divine Comedy*.

- **Elijah:** Meaning "the Lord is my God" in Hebrew, Elijah honors a powerful biblical prophet known for his faith and miracles. This enduring name represents devotion, strength, and a lasting spiritual legacy.

- **Ephraim:** A Hebrew name meaning "fruitful," Ephraim symbolizes productivity and blessings as one of the founders of the twelve tribes of Israel. Unique yet rooted in tradition, it inspires meaningful living.

- **Esther:** Of Persian origin, meaning "star," Esther celebrates a heroic biblical figure who saved her people through wisdom and bravery. It embodies strength and justice.

- **Ignacio:** A Spanish name derived from Latin *Ignatius*, meaning "fiery" or "ardent," Ignacio reflects passion and energy, tied to Saint Ignatius of Loyola. Its unique and elegant tone ensures cultural and spiritual depth.

- **Isaiah:** A Hebrew name meaning "salvation of the Lord," Isaiah celebrates a compassionate prophet who brought messages of hope and redemption, symbolizing faith and resilience.

- **Joan:** A Hebrew name meaning "God is gracious," Joan carries a rich legacy through figures like Joan of Arc. It represents resilience, faith, and courage intertwined with a sense of divine purpose.

- **Malia:** A Hawaiian name meaning "calm" or "peaceful," Malia reflects grace and serenity. It is also a variant of Maria, linking it to biblical and cultural roots. Malia's soothing tone and elegant charm give it global appeal.

- **Martin:** Of Latin origin, meaning "dedicated to Mars," Martin symbolizes bravery and strength. Its historical ties to leaders like Martin Luther King Jr. add depth and inspiration. Martin's simplicity and global usage make it a classic choice.

- **Mateo:** A Spanish variant of Matthew, meaning "gift of God," Mateo is a timeless name with warmth and charm. It is beloved across cultures for its connection to gratitude and faith.

- **Miriam:** Meaning "wished-for child" or "sea of bitterness" in Hebrew, Miriam honors Moses's courageous sister. It symbolizes love, devotion, and the joy a child brings.

- **Mohammed:** Of Arabic origin, meaning "praiseworthy," Mohammed honors Prophet Muhammad and reflects moral excellence, spiritual devotion, and inspiration.

- **Nicholas:** A Greek name meaning "victory of the people," Nicholas reflects leadership and generosity. Tied to Saint Nicholas, it carries spiritual and cultural significance. Nicholas's versatility is enriched by nicknames like Nick and Nico.

- **Omar:** Of Arabic origin, meaning "flourishing" or "eloquent," Omar exudes strength and wisdom. It has historical significance through figures like Omar Khayyam and Caliph Omar. Omar's simplicity and cultural depth make it a timeless choice.

- **Rania:** Of Arabic origin, meaning "queen" or "gazing," Rania carries a regal and poetic quality. It reflects strength and grace, making it a majestic and meaningful name.

- **Santiago:** A Spanish name meaning "Saint James," Santiago honors the patron saint of Spain and reflects a strong cultural and spiritual heritage, symbolizing devotion and perseverance.

- **Sebastian:** A Latin name meaning "venerable" or "revered," Sebastian carries a dignified tone. It is tied to Saint Sebastian, the patron saint of athletes, symbolizing resilience and faith. Sebastian's elegance and international appeal make it a sophisticated classic.

- **Simon:** Of Hebrew and Greek origin, Simon means "to hear" or "listening." Associated with Simon Peter, one of Jesus's apostles, it embodies intelligence, thoughtfulness, and timeless faith.

- **Solomon:** Of Hebrew origin, meaning "peace," the name Solomon is celebrated for its association with wisdom and leadership, honoring the biblical king renowned for his fair judgments and enduring legacy of knowledge and understanding.

- **Stephanie:** Of Greek origin, meaning "crown" or "garland," Stephanie symbolizes honor and victory. It is tied to Saint Stephen, reflecting spiritual and historical significance. Stephanie's graceful tone and versatility ensure its timeless appeal.

- **Theresa:** Derived from Greek, meaning "summer" or "to harvest," Theresa reflects vitality and growth and is celebrated through figures like Saint Teresa of Avila and Mother Teresa.

- **Timothy:** A Greek name meaning "honoring God," Timothy carries spiritual and historical significance. It is tied to the biblical companion of Saint Paul, symbolizing faith and devotion. Timothy's approachable sound and enduring charm make it a beloved choice.

- **Valentino:** An Italian name meaning "strong" or "healthy," Valentino symbolizes love and vitality. Its romantic and elegant sound is tied to Saint Valentine. Valentino's flair and charm ensure its enduring popularity.

Names tied to historical and religious figures carry legacies of strength, faith, and moral integrity that resonate across time. Whether honoring prophets, saints, or leaders, these names connect your child to stories of courage, wisdom, and perseverance.

Cultural Names That Honor Heritage and Tradition

In previous chapters, we explored classic, rare, and even gender-neutral names that celebrate individuality and creativity, often drawing inspiration from cultural traditions. Now, let's go discuss how cultural names celebrate family roots, preserving a connection to heritage and passing down stories, values, and traditions. These names are bridges between the past and present, serving as reminders of identity and pride.

Here are a few examples:

- **Akira:** Of Japanese origin, meaning "bright" or "intelligent," Akira symbolizes brilliance and resilience. Its multicultural roots make it a dynamic choice for a child destined to shine.

- **Amani:** A name of Arabic and Swahili origins, meaning "wishes" or "peace," Amani reflects hope and tranquility. It's a beautiful choice for parents who value harmony and aspire to a peaceful future.

- **Amina:** An Arabic name meaning "safe one" or "faithful," Amina reflects integrity and kindness. Revered in Muslim communities, it honors Prophet Muhammad's mother and represents a legacy of trust and faith.

- **Anjali:** A Sanskrit name meaning "divine offering," Anjali reflects reverence and devotion. Associated with spiritual greetings in Hindu and Buddhist traditions, it embodies grace and heritage.

- **Ariana:** Derived from Greek and Welsh origins, Ariana means "most holy" and "silver." Related to Ariadne, it conveys purity and preciousness, offering an ethereal and cherished quality.

- **Aurelio:** Of Latin origin, meaning "golden," Aurelio symbolizes brilliance and artistry. Derived from the Roman Aurelius, it celebrates intellect, warmth, and enduring ideals and has the feminine variant Aurelia.

- **Ava:** With Latin, Hebrew, and Persian origins, Ava means "bird," "life," and "voice." Its connections to freedom, vitality, and lyrical beauty make it a timeless and energetic choice.

- **Brianna:** An Irish name derived from Brian, meaning "high" or "noble," Brianna reflects strength and beauty. Its melodic tone gives it a feminine yet empowering quality. Brianna's modern charm and cultural roots make it a popular choice.

- **Bruno:** Of Germanic origin, meaning "brown" or "armor," Bruno reflects strength and resilience. Its bold, short sound gives it a modern, edgy vibe with historical roots. Bruno's uniqueness and cultural versatility make it a standout name.

- **Cian:** Of Irish origin, meaning "ancient" or "enduring one," Cian is tied to mythology and the god of healing. It represents resilience and Celtic heritage with heroic undertones.

- **Ebele:** An Igbo name from Nigeria, meaning "compassion" or "mercy," Ebele reflects kindness, warmth, and emotional depth. Its cultural uniqueness and meaningful tone make it a rare and beautiful choice.

- **Eloise:** A French name meaning "healthy" or "wide," this name's medieval origins tie it to Saint Héloïse, a renowned scholar, adding historical resonance. Its melodic sound and association with intelligence and creativity make it a timeless choice.

- **Farah:** A name of Arabic origin, meaning "joy" or "happiness," Farah embodies positivity and celebration. Its simplicity and elegance make it a bright and uplifting choice.

- **Hana:** A name with diverse origins, meaning "happiness" or "flower," Hana represents joy and beauty. It spans traditions from the Old Testament to Hawaiian culture, offering universal appeal.

- **Hiroshi:** A Japanese name meaning "tolerant" or "prosperous," Hiroshi embodies kindness and grace. Reflecting selfless hospitality, it inspires generosity and compassion, resonating with cultural depth.

- **Idris:** Of Arabic origin, Idris means "interpreter" or "studious." In Islamic tradition, Idris is a prophet, adding spiritual significance. Its rare and lyrical tone makes it a standout name with cultural depth.

- **Imani:** Of Arabic and Swahili origins, meaning "faith," Imani inspires trust and optimism. It symbolizes inner strength and spiritual connection, particularly in Eastern African cultures.

- **Indira:** Of Sanskrit origin, meaning "beauty" and "splendor," Indira is linked to the Hindu goddess Lakshmi and symbolizes prosperity and luck. Associated with Indira Gandhi, it exudes strength, elegance, and leadership.

- **Inez:** Of Portuguese and Spanish origin, meaning "pure" or "chaste," Inez is associated with Saint Agnes, reflecting spirituality and faith, with a refined elegance rooted in European tradition.

- **Ishaan:** A Sanskrit name meaning "sun" or "lord," Ishaan carries spiritual and cultural depth. It is associated with vitality, brightness, and divine energy in Hindu tradition. Its melodic sound and rich heritage ensure its lasting appeal.

- **Jocelyn:** Of Old French origin meaning "member of the Gauts tribe," Jocelyn carries historical depth. It balances sophistication and warmth, with a timeless and approachable feel. Jocelyn's adaptability across cultures ensures its lasting popularity.

- **Kendrick:** Of Old English and Welsh origin, Kendrick means "royal power" or "champion." It reflects strength and leadership, with a modern, commanding tone. Kendrick's versatility makes it a bold and dynamic choice.

- **Kwame:** Of Akan origin, meaning "born on Saturday," Kwame is a culturally rich name that holds special significance in Ghanaian traditions, symbolizing identity and heritage.

- **Layla:** An Arabic name meaning "night," Layla evokes mystery and beauty, often celebrated in poetry and song. Its lyrical charm has made it a beloved choice across cultures.

- **Leonardo:** A Germanic name meaning "lion-hearted," Leonardo symbolizes strength and courage. Popular in Italy and Spain, its artistic and historical ties, like those to Leonardo da Vinci, enhance its cultural richness. The modern variant Leo offers a bold, succinct alternative.

- **Lila:** Multicultural in origin, Lila means "night" in Arabic and "divine play" in Sanskrit. Its Persian ties to the lilac tree evoke tranquility and beauty, making it a vibrant, creative choice.

- **Malachi:** A Hebrew name meaning "messenger of God," it is associated with the prophet Malachi and Irish traditions. Malachi blends spiritual depth and adaptability, offering timeless appeal.

- **Malik:** Of Arabic origin, meaning "king," Malik conveys strength, authority, and leadership. Its regal tone is complemented by its spiritual significance in Islamic tradition. Malik's simplicity and cultural resonance make it a powerful, timeless name.

- **Marcelo:** A Spanish and Portuguese name derived from Latin *Marcellus*, meaning "young warrior," Marcelo carries a sophisticated and elegant tone with historical resonance. Its international appeal makes it a versatile and distinguished choice.

- **Priya:** Of Sanskrit origin, meaning "beloved" or "dear," Priya is a classic Indian name that carries warmth and affection, symbolizing love and cherished connections.

- **Rami:** Of Arabic and Hebrew origins, meaning "archer" or "elevated," Rami is a name that conveys direction and ambition, rooted in both cultural and biblical significance.

- **Ravi:** A Sanskrit name meaning "sun," Ravi symbolizes vitality, brilliance, and life. In Hindu culture, it represents energy and divine connection. Ravi's simplicity and rich cultural significance make it a radiant and enduring choice.

- **Renata:** Of Latin origin, meaning "reborn," Renata symbolizes renewal and vitality, drawing on its historical and spiritual connections for an uplifting and meaningful choice.

- **Rohan:** A Sanskrit and Irish name, meaning "ascending" or "red-haired," Rohan blends cultural versatility with an adventurous spirit, making it a strong and dynamic choice.

- **Saanvi:** Saanvi, an Indian name tied to the goddess Lakshmi, symbolizes spiritual connection and ambition. It conveys meanings like "summit" or "following," blending reverence and determination.

- **Scarlett:** Of French origin, meaning "red," Scarlett evokes passion, joy, and courage. Popularized by Scarlett O'Hara, it reflects vibrancy and history, fitting for a spirited individual.

- **Suki:** A Japanese name meaning "beloved" or "loved one," Suki reflects warmth and joy, combining its endearing nature with a universally simple and cherished charm.

- **Tariq:** An Arabic name meaning "visitor" or "morning star," Tariq signifies arrival and light, drawing on celestial imagery and cultural heritage, with a connection to guidance and inspiration.

- **Valentina:** A Latin name meaning "strong" or "healthy," Valentina symbolizes love and resilience. Tied to Saint Valentine, it reflects hope, strength, and a life filled with affection.

- **Yara:** With Arabic and Brazilian roots, meaning "small butterfly" or "water lady," Yara is tied to mythology and strength. Its enchanting and cross-cultural charm makes it unique.

- **Zola:** With African and Latin origins, meaning "peace" or "earth," Zola is a vibrant and distinctive name, celebrating harmony and grounded individuality with global cultural roots.

Cultural names are vessels of history, identity, and pride. By choosing a name with deep roots in heritage and tradition, you give your child a gift that connects them to their ancestry and the values that define your family.

Wrapping Up

Spiritual, biblical, and cultural names connect children to their roots, reflecting values, traditions, and histories that transcend generations. These names carry profound meanings, serving as anchors of identity and guiding principles for a meaningful life. They honor the past while empowering children to forge their own paths with confidence and purpose.

In the next chapter, we'll explore names inspired by places and travel, evoking wonder, discovery, and a sense of adventure. Let's embark on a journey into names that inspire a love for the world and its stories!

Chapter 7:
Names Inspired by Places and Travel

Every corner of the world holds a story, and some of those stories become part of our own personal journeys. Whether it's a city where you experienced life-changing moments, a natural wonder that left you breathless, or a destination that inspires dreams of adventure, places uniquely shape our identities. Names inspired by places and travel capture that magic, offering a sense of location and an invitation to explore, connect, and dream.

In this chapter, we'll learn how place-inspired names allow you to share your love for the world with your child. From names that honor personal milestones and cultural heritage to those that evoke wanderlust and individuality, place names carry many meanings. They can celebrate a favorite destination, embody the spirit of adventure, or offer your child a distinctive identity that sets them apart.

Let's explore the map of inspiration and uncover a name that's just as extraordinary as the places that inspire it.

Personal and Emotional Connections to Place Names

For many, place-inspired names carry deep emotional significance. They may commemorate where life-changing moments occurred, like a first meeting, a honeymoon, or a place of peace. A name like Vienna, the "City of Music," embodies romance and inspiration, while Dublin ties to Ireland's rich culture.

Place names also celebrate cultural heritage. Parents might choose India or Geneva to reflect ancestral pride or honor family roots. These names become bridges between generations, keeping traditions alive and connecting children to their origins. Additionally, they can embody the qualities of a place: Geneva suggests peace and diplomacy, while Ronan signifies strength and resilience.

These names often carry symbolic meaning beyond geography, capturing the emotional landscapes of life. Whether tied to a small town, a bustling city, or a distant land, they preserve memories and create enduring legacies of love and connection.

Let's explore some of those names:

- **Austin:** A Latin name meaning "great" or "majestic," Austin exudes strength and creativity. Associated with Austin, Texas, a hub of music and innovation, this classic yet contemporary name remains enduringly popular.

- **Chelsea:** Derived from Old English, meaning "landing place for chalk," Chelsea reflects calm sophistication. Its cultural ties to the London neighborhood add to its modern allure. Chelsea's timeless charm and sleek sound make it a beloved unisex name.

- **Dublin:** Inspired by Ireland's capital city and derived from Dubh Linn meaning "black pool," this name connects to the city's rich culture and adventurous spirit. A distinctive choice, Dublin reflects individuality and a love for history.

- **Florence:** Of Latin origin, meaning "blossoming" or "flourishing," Florence symbolizes growth and prosperity. Tied to Florence Nightingale and the Renaissance city of Florence, Italy, this timeless name reflects art, history, and progress.

- **Geneva:** A German name meaning "juniper tree" or "bending river," this name also references the elegant Swiss city. Its ties to nature and the juniper tree's protective symbolism add depth to this thoughtful and charming choice.

- **Haven:** Derived from Old English, meaning "harbor" or "safe place," this name symbolizes comfort and security. Popularized by its modern appeal, Haven is ideal for parents seeking a name reflecting love, warmth, and sanctuary.

- **India:** Of Latin and Sanskrit origin, meaning "from the Indus River," India represents the cultural and geographic richness of South Asia. This name inspires exploration and resilience, offering timeless global appeal.

- **Kingston:** An English name meaning "king's town," Kingston combines regal sophistication with contemporary flair. It is also tied to the vibrant capital of Jamaica, offering cultural richness and a spirited vibe.

- **London:** Of uncertain origin, London is believed to derive from the Celtic name *Londinium,* possibly meaning "wild" or "bold." As the name of England's vibrant capital, London embodies a blend of historical depth and modern sophistication.

- **Lourdes:** Of French origin, meaning "craggy slope," Lourdes is associated with the Marian shrine in southern France, known for its spiritual significance and miracles. This elegant and sacred name reflects faith and devotion.

- **Memphis:** A name of Greek and Egyptian origin, meaning "enduring beauty," Memphis is associated with the ancient Egyptian capital and the lively city in Tennessee. This name embodies history, culture, and a modern sense of artistry.

- **Nara:** Nara, a Japanese city, means "oak" or "peaceful" in Japanese and "happy" in Celtic origins. Rich in cultural and historical significance, this name reflects serenity and strength. Its minimalistic and global charm makes it a rare and versatile choice.

- **Odessa:** A name of Greek origin, meaning "long journey," this name is associated with the Ukrainian port city on the Black Sea. With ties to mythology and adventure, Odessa embodies resilience and charm, offering a unique choice for a child with a love for exploration.

- **Paris:** Of Greek origin, meaning "wallet" or "pouch," Paris is famously tied to the romantic French capital and the Trojan prince in Greek mythology. This elegant name carries historical and cultural significance, making it a sophisticated and timeless option.

- **Remy:** Of French origin, meaning "from Rheims" or "oarsman," this name reflects sophistication and determination. Rooted in history and culture, it also carries modern appeal with playful ties to Ratatouille's chef.

- **Rhodes:** A Greek island steeped in mythology and history, Rhodes symbolizes strength and beauty. It also refers to the Colossus of Rhodes, one of the Seven Wonders of the Ancient World.

- **Ronan:** An Irish name meaning "little seal," Ronan connects to Celtic mythology and the sea. With ties to Irish saints and a love for nature, Ronan is a melodic and timeless name full of character.

- **Savannah:** Of Spanish and Native American origin, meaning "from the open plain," Savannah symbolizes openness and exploration. Referencing Savannah, Georgia, this name embodies Southern charm and a love for nature.

- **Siena:** An Italian name meaning "from Siena," this name captures the charm of the historic Tuscan city, renowned for its rich history and vibrant culture. It also reflects the orange-red hue inspired by the city, symbolizing creativity and wanderlust.

- **Valencia:** A Spanish name meaning "bravery" or "strength," it is also the name of a vibrant Mediterranean city in Spain. Valencia combines elegance with energy, reflecting beauty, courage, and a connection to Spanish culture.

- **Verona:** Of Italian origin, meaning "truth" or "spring," this name is tied to the city of Verona, renowned as the setting for Shakespeare's *Romeo and Juliet*. Verona exudes romance and timeless beauty, making it a poetic and enchanting choice.

- **Vienna:** A Latin name meaning "city in Austria," Vienna honors the cultural brilliance of Vienna, the "City of Music," home to classical composers like Mozart. It also nods to the iconic Billy Joel song, making it a sophisticated and artistic choice.

Place-inspired names offer a unique opportunity to celebrate your ancestry or a destination that symbolizes adventure and resilience.

Place Names That Evoke a Sense of Adventure and Wanderlust

While some place-inspired names are rooted in personal memories or cultural heritage, others speak to the thrill of discovery and the allure of the unknown. These names invite a sense of adventure, curiosity, and a love for exploration. For parents who dream of a life filled with worldly experiences and open horizons for their child, choosing a name tied to far-off places or iconic landmarks can be a way to inspire a spirit of wanderlust.

Names like Cairo, Rio, and Everest evoke images of distant lands and extraordinary adventures. Whether the vibrant energy of a bustling city, the natural grandeur of a towering peak, or the rhythmic allure of a legendary river, these names encapsulate the spirit of movement and exploration. They're perfect for parents who see life as a journey and want their children to embrace the world with wonder and bravery.

Examples might include:

- **Alaska:** A name of Aleut origin, meaning "great land," Alaska evokes the rugged beauty and vast wilderness of the U.S. state. This bold and adventurous name symbolizes exploration, resilience, and connection to nature.

- **Anden:** A Scandinavian name meaning "spirit" or "breath," Anden conveys vitality and creativity. Its connection to the Andes mountain range adds grandeur and natural beauty, making it a distinctive and inspiring name.

- **Brooklyn:** A gender-neutral name with German, Dutch, and British origins, meaning "small stream" or "land by the brook," it also reflects the creative energy of New York's borough. Brooklyn celebrates individuality and artistic expression.

- **Byron:** Of Old English origin, meaning "barn for cows," Byron is celebrated for its literary ties to the romantic poet Lord Byron. This refined and creative name carries a sense of artistry and intellect, ideal for a child with a poetic spirit.

- **Cairo:** Of Egyptian and Arabic origin, meaning "the strong" or "the victorious," Cairo reflects strength and cultural heritage. Named after Egypt's bustling capital, it symbolizes resilience and triumph, inspired by the city's ties to Mars and its historical significance.

- **Carson:** Of Scottish and Irish origin, meaning "son of Carr," Carson is a gender-neutral name that conveys strength and resilience. Its modern usage reflects adventure and reliability, making it a versatile and enduring choice.

- **Cheyenne:** Of Native American origin, this name refers to the indigenous Cheyenne people and their language. It is also tied to the capital of Wyoming, symbolizing resilience and cultural richness. With its strong and melodic tone, Cheyenne evokes both history and natural beauty.

- **Dakota:** A gender-neutral name of Native American Sioux origin, meaning "friend" or "ally," Dakota embodies loyalty, bravery, and artistry. Its unisex appeal and connection to the community make it an empowering and versatile choice.

- **Denver:** An English name meaning "green valley," Denver is also the capital of Colorado, known for its mountainous landscapes and adventurous spirit. This strong and modern name symbolizes nature, resilience, and exploration.

- **Everest:** Of British origin, meaning "dweller on the Eure River," this name also honors Mount Everest, the world's tallest peak. Symbolizing strength and achievement, Everest inspires perseverance and reaching great heights in life.

- **Havana:** A Spanish name meaning "of the Habana people," this name honors Cuba's capital with roots in indigenous culture and history. Havana blends cultural richness and historical depth, offering a unique and meaningful choice.

- **Jackson:** An English name meaning "son of Jack," Jackson is a strong and popular choice with ties to historical figures like Michael Jackson. It blends tradition with modern appeal, offering a name that conveys leadership and reliability.

- **Orlando:** A name of Italian origin, meaning "famous land," Orlando is associated with Florida's lively city and Shakespeare's *As You Like It*. It combines charm and strength, making it a dynamic and classic name choice.

- **Rio:** A gender-neutral Spanish name meaning "river," Rio evokes flowing water and vibrant energy. Associated with the Brazilian city Rio de Janeiro, known for its lively Carnival, this nature-inspired name celebrates life, color, and movement.

- **Sydney:** Of French and British origins, meaning "Saint Denis" or "dweller by the well-watered land," it connects to the vibrant Australian city and Saint-Denis, the patron saint of Paris. Sydney combines spiritual and worldly inspiration with a touch of creativity.

- **Tahoe:** A name of Native American origin, meaning "big water," Tahoe is tied to the picturesque lake spanning California and Nevada. This nature-inspired name reflects tranquility, adventure, and a love for the outdoors.

Place-inspired names symbolize the values of adaptability, strength, and a love for discovery, making them perfect for parents who wish to spark a sense of wonder in their child's heart.

Unique and Distinctive Nature of Place-Based Names

Place-inspired names offer an exceptional opportunity for parents to give their child a name that feels truly one-of-a-kind. Unlike more commonly used place names, unique and distinctive choices stand out for their rarity and originality, providing a sense of individuality that resonates with parents who value uniqueness. They carry an air of intrigue, often sparking curiosity and inviting meaningful stories about the places they represent.

For some, these names are a way to express a passion for global exploration or admiration for a specific culture or region. Distinctive place names also offer a sense of timelessness unbound by fleeting trends, ensuring that the name remains as unique as the individual it represents. Additionally, these names can feel like a blank canvas, encouraging the child to define their identity while carrying the inspiration of a remarkable place.

- **Avalon:** Of Celtic origin, meaning "island of apples," Avalon is tied to Arthurian legend as a place of paradise and healing. This enchanting name exudes magic, mystery, and timeless beauty, making it a captivating choice.

- **Blair:** A name of Scottish origin, meaning "field" or "plain," Blair is a gender-neutral choice associated with strength and sophistication. Its ties to nature and its sleek sound make it a modern and versatile option.

- **Calais:** A gender-neutral name of Greek origin, meaning "changing color," it also references the French port city known for its historical significance. Calais offers mystery and versatility, making it a distinctive and meaningful name.

- **Delphi:** Of Greek origin, meaning "hollow" or "womb," Delphi is associated with the Oracle of Delphi, a sacred site in ancient Greece. This mystical name carries a sense of wisdom, spirituality, and history, making it both unique and inspiring.

- **Devon:** Of English origin, meaning "defender," or referencing the Devon region, this name is sleek and contemporary. Its clean, versatile sound makes it a popular gender-neutral choice. Devon offers a perfect mix of geographic charm and modern appeal.

- **Holland:** A name of Dutch origin, meaning "wooded land," it is associated with the Netherlands, a country known for its tulip fields, windmills, and artistic legacy. Holland offers a fresh, worldly feel and is a versatile choice for parents inspired by travel and cultural charm.

- **Kyoto:** A city-based name of Japanese origin, meaning "capital," this name reflects Kyoto's historical role as Japan's capital for over a millennium. Its cultural significance and connection to Japan's history make it a refined and meaningful choice.

- **Marbella:** Linked to the Spanish coastal city, this name derives from the Arabic *Marbal·la*, meaning "fertile district." Marbella's association with luxurious beaches and Mediterranean charm makes it a sophisticated and culturally rich choice.

- **Marietta:** Of Italian origin, this name is a diminutive of Maria, meaning "bitter" or "beloved." It draws inspiration from the charming city of Marietta, Georgia, reflecting Southern elegance. With its vintage sound and geographic connection, Marietta carries timeless warmth.

- **Milan:** Of Slavic origin, meaning "gracious" or "dear," this gender-neutral name also represents Italy's fashion capital. Milan combines warmth with elegance, making it a stylish and heartfelt choice for parents inspired by grace and sophistication.

- **Monroe:** Of Scottish origin, meaning "mouth of the river," Monroe is a strong, gender-neutral name with historic ties to U.S. President James Monroe and cultural associations with Marilyn

Monroe. It combines elegance with strength, offering timeless appeal.

- **Montana:** Of Latin origin, meaning "mountain," this gender-neutral name evokes strength, adventure, and natural beauty. Associated with the U.S. state known for its breathtaking landscapes, Montana is ideal for nature-loving parents seeking a grounding, resilient name.

- **Oslo:** An Old Norse name meaning "estuary" or "meadow of the gods," Oslo connects to Norway's capital and its Norse mythology. This gender-neutral choice blends Scandinavian culture with modern elegance and a touch of mystery.

- **Petra:** A name of Greek origin, meaning "rock," Petra is tied to the ancient Jordanian city known for its breathtaking architecture and archaeological significance. This strong and timeless name symbolizes resilience and cultural depth.

- **Sahara:** Derived from the Arabic *Ṣaḥrā*, meaning "desert," this name captures the vast beauty and mystery of the Sahara Desert. With its golden imagery and ties to Sarah, meaning "princess," Sahara blends natural splendor with a regal touch.

- **Salem:** Of Hebrew origin, meaning "peace," Salem is tied to the biblical city of Jerusalem and the historic New England town. This serene and spiritual name reflects harmony and carries cultural depth and timeless appeal.

- **Tahiti:** A Polynesian name meaning "little king Hiro," this name is tied to the stunning island in French Polynesia known for its natural beauty and vibrant culture. Tahiti offers a unique, exotic name imbued with mythology and tropical splendor.

- **Zurich:** Derived from the Latin *Turicum*, meaning "belonging to Tūros," this name represents Switzerland's largest city, a center of finance and culture. Zurich offers sophistication and a link to Swiss heritage, making it a worldly and distinctive option.

Unique and distinctive place-based names offer parents a chance to give their children a name that is as rare and extraordinary as the locations that inspire them.

Wrapping Up

While this chapter has highlighted an array of names inspired by places and travel, the true beauty of place-based names lies in their ability to reflect personal meaning. Whether it's a bustling city, a serene natural wonder, or a location tied to a cherished memory, the possibilities are endless. As parents, you have the opportunity to draw inspiration from the places that have shaped your journey, selecting a name that resonates with your unique experiences and values.

As we conclude our exploration of names inspired by places, it's time to bring everything together. In the next and final chapter, we'll offer practical tips and thoughtful guidance to help you navigate the naming process with confidence. Let's move forward and discover the final steps to choosing the perfect name!

Chapter 8:
Final Tips for Choosing the Right Name

As you approach the end of this journey, you may feel both excitement and a bit of pressure. Choosing the right name is no small task—it's a deeply personal decision that will resonate for a lifetime. Throughout this guide, we've explored key dimensions of naming: cultural and family ties, practicality, social perception, and the meaning behind names. Now, it's time to bring all these insights together.

This chapter is about helping you reflect on the process, refine your choices, and finalize a name that feels meaningful and timeless. Remember, the "perfect" name isn't about meeting every criterion; it's about finding the one that feels right for your child and family. These final tips will guide you to a confident decision that reflects your hopes and values.

How the Name Pairs With the Last Name

A name's flow with the last name is a practical and aesthetic consideration. The sound of a full name can influence how it feels, how easily it is remembered, and how well it resonates in different settings. Here are some things to consider:

- **Say the full name aloud:** Hearing the name aloud helps you evaluate its rhythm and identify any awkward transitions. For example, names like Mia Anderson might blend into "Mianderson" when spoken quickly, while names such as Lucas Carter have a natural cadence. Saying the name in different tones and contexts can reveal whether it sounds smooth and cohesive.

- **Balance syllables:** Balancing the length of the first name with the last name often creates a pleasing rhythm. Short first names like Eli or Anna pair well with longer surnames, while longer first names like Alexander or Isabella often match better with shorter last names. A well-matched syllable balance enhances the name's flow and harmony.

- **Avoid unintended rhymes:** Watch out for rhymes or repetitive sounds that could create unintended humor. Names like Harry Barry or Lilly Milly might seem playful but could lead to teasing. Similarly, names like Justin Case or Ben Dover should be avoided to prevent inadvertent wordplay.

- **Check the initials:** Writing out initials is an easy way to avoid problematic acronyms. For instance, initials like CAT (Caden Anthony Taylor) or BIB (Bryan Isaac Bennett) might lead to unwanted associations. Ensuring the initials don't spell something distracting helps avoid future embarrassment.

- **Hyphenated or unique last names:** If your child will have a hyphenated surname or an uncommon last name, shorter first names often work best. For example, Hal Holden-Bach feels balanced, whereas Elizabeth Holden-Bach might feel overly lengthy. Testing the full name aloud ensures it feels natural and manageable in daily use.

Think About Nicknames

Nicknames are often a natural extension of a given name, evolving organically over time. Anticipating potential nicknames helps ensure they align with your preferences and fit well with the last name.

- **Common nicknames:** Some names naturally shorten, like Benjamin to Ben or Katherine to Kate. Consider how these variations might feel in casual or professional settings. For instance, Theodore might become Teddy, which feels informal, while Madeline might shorten to Maddie, giving it a youthful tone.

- **Unexpected nicknames:** Unique or longer names may lead to creative nicknames. For example, Aurora might become Rory, and Sebastian could turn into Seb. These variations often arise from family or peers, so it's helpful to think about whether you're comfortable with potential outcomes.

- **Nicknames with the last name:** Test how nicknames sound with the last name. For instance, William Johnson shortening to Will Johnson sounds polished, while Isabella Turner becoming Izzy Turner feels playful. Pairing potential nicknames with the last name ensures they maintain harmony.

Test the Name in Sentences

Beyond saying the full name aloud, testing it in conversational phrases can help you determine how it feels in everyday use. This practical step reveals subtleties that might not be apparent otherwise.

Try phrases like:

- "Hi, I'm [Name]."
- "This is my friend, [Name]."
- "Can I speak to [Name]?"

Hearing the name in context allows you to evaluate its tone, flow, and ease of use. A name like Sophia Carter might feel elegant and smooth, while Alexandria Bennet may come across as more formal or require a nickname for casual settings. Testing names in real-life scenarios helps you choose one that feels intuitive and natural.

Consider Popularity

A name's popularity can influence how it's perceived and how unique it feels. Popular names like Emma or Liam have broad appeal but might be shared with many peers, while less common names can offer individuality.

- **Evaluating trends:** Online tools and baby name statistics, like those on The Bump website, make it easy to see a name's ranking and popularity trends. For example, parents drawn to Emma for its timeless charm might discover its frequent use and opt for a less common alternative like Emmeline (Barrett, 2010).

- **Balancing familiarity and uniqueness:** Names further down popularity lists often strike a balance between recognition and individuality. Variations of popular names, such as Elena instead of Ella, can add a personal touch while maintaining appeal.

- **Pop culture influence:** Some names rise sharply due to media or pop culture but may fade over time. For instance, names inspired by movies or celebrities might feel trendy now but lose their appeal later. Conversely, timeless names like Elizabeth or James remain consistent in popularity without feeling tied to a specific trend.

- **Regional variations:** A name's popularity can vary by region. A name that's common nationally might be less so in your local area, providing uniqueness without straying far from familiar territory.

Reflecting on popularity helps you decide whether you prefer a name that stands out or blends in, ensuring it aligns with your family's priorities.

Sleep on It

Choosing a name is one of the most meaningful decisions you'll make as a parent, but it can also feel overwhelming. If you find yourself stuck or unsure, taking a step back is often the best solution. Naming your child is a journey, not a race, and giving yourself permission to pause can bring clarity and calm to the process.

Stepping away allows your mind to rest and reset. After some time, you may find that a particular name resonates more deeply, or you'll gain a clearer sense of which options feel right. Consider taking a day or two—or even longer if needed—to reflect without overanalyzing. Let the possibilities rest in the back of your mind while you focus on other tasks. When you revisit your list, certain names may stand out more, or your perspective on some options might shift.

This simple act of "sleeping on it" is a valuable tool for narrowing your choices and approaching the decision with fresh eyes. Taking your time ensures that the name you choose reflects your intentions, allowing you to move forward with confidence and ease.

Imagine How They Will Share the Name's Story

Every name has a story, and imagining how your child will share theirs can add a meaningful layer to your choice. Think about the moment you'll explain why you picked their name. Whether it's rooted in family history, cultural tradition, or personal inspiration, this story can connect your child to their identity and values.

Ask yourself: What do I want my child to feel when they hear their name's story? For example, choosing Amelia to represent courage and independence, inspired by Amelia Earhart, gives your child a narrative tied to qualities you hope they'll embody. Alternatively, a name like Noah might honor a grandparent or reflect spiritual beliefs. These connections create a sense of belonging and purpose.

Even if the name was chosen simply because it brought you joy, that's a story worth sharing too. "We picked your name because it made us happy every time we said it" is a heartfelt explanation your child can cherish throughout their life.

Consider how the story of the name might evolve. Will it inspire curiosity about family roots, cultural heritage, or historical figures? Will it reflect values or dreams you hold for your child? Visualizing these conversations helps confirm your decision and ensures the name feels intentional.

Involve Siblings in the Process

Including siblings in the naming process is a wonderful way to create a sense of connection and excitement within your family. When older children are involved, they feel valued and invested in welcoming the new baby.

Siblings of different ages can participate in various ways. Younger children might enjoy suggesting playful or creative names, even if their ideas are whimsical. Suggestions like Princess Sparkle or Superhero Steve bring humor and joy to the process. Older siblings might prefer helping to narrow down the final list or voting on their favorites, offering meaningful input while learning about the importance of naming.

This involvement also provides opportunities to share family traditions or explain the significance of certain names. For instance, you could discuss why a particular name honors a relative or reflects your cultural heritage. These conversations help siblings understand the thoughtfulness behind the decision, fostering a sense of pride and connection.

When siblings help choose the name, they are more likely to feel ownership and excitement about the new addition to the family. Imagine the joy of an older sibling proudly telling friends, "I helped pick my baby sister's name!" This collaborative approach strengthens family bonds and sets the stage for a positive, inclusive dynamic.

While their input is valuable, it's important to manage expectations. Gently explain that while their ideas are appreciated, the final decision rests with you as parents. This ensures they feel heard while maintaining your authority to choose the name that best fits your family.

Let Go of Perfection

The search for the "perfect" name can feel daunting, but the truth is that no name is flawless. Every name carries unique qualities, and no single choice can cover every scenario, appeal to everyone, or guarantee universal approval. Instead of striving for unattainable perfection, focus on finding a name that feels meaningful and aligned with your family's values and story.

Ask yourself: Does the name reflect the qualities or traditions you want to honor? Does it resonate with you and your partner as something your child will carry with pride? These considerations are far more important than aiming for a name that meets an impossible standard.

Remember, names grow with the people who carry them. A name that feels ordinary today might take on extraordinary meaning as your child builds their life and legacy. Similarly, a name's significance deepens over time as it becomes entwined with memories and experiences.

It's also okay if not everyone loves your choice. What matters most is that the name feels right to you. Trust your instincts—they are guided by the love and thoughtfulness you're putting into this decision.

By letting go of the pressure for perfection, you can focus on what truly matters: giving your child a name that feels intentional and heartfelt. The right name doesn't need to tick every box—it simply needs to feel like a meaningful gift of love and connection.

Wrapping Up

Choosing a name is a deeply personal decision that reflects your family's story, values, and dreams. Trusting your instincts and the emotional connection you feel to a name is key. While outside opinions can provide perspective, they shouldn't overshadow what feels right in your heart. Parents who choose names based on personal meaning often find lasting satisfaction, even if their choice diverges from popular trends.

As you reflect on these tips and ideas, remember that naming is part of a larger journey. The right name will become a cherished part of your child's identity, a foundation for their story, and a testament to the care and thought you've put into this moment.

Take your time, trust yourself, and enjoy the process. Whatever name you choose, it will be a beautiful start to your child's unique life.

Chapter 9: Baby Name List

Boy Names

1. Aarav 48
   - **Meaning:** "peaceful" or "calm"
   - **Description:** Of Sanskrit origin, Aarav signifies serenity and wisdom, reflecting a harmonious and strong character
   - **Chapter:** 3

2. Aaron...18
   - **Meaning:** "exalted" or "high mountain"
   - **Description:** A Hebrew name with biblical significance, Aaron was the brother of Moses and a symbol of leadership and strength.
   - **Chapter:** 2

3. Abel 114
   - **Meaning:** "breath" or "vapor"
   - **Description:** A Hebrew name associated with the biblical figure Abel, symbolizing humility and devotion.
   - **Chapter:** 6

4. Abraham..122

- **Meaning:** "high father" or "father of multitudes"
- **Description:** A Hebrew name associated with the biblical patriarch, symbolizing leadership, faith, and wisdom.
- **Chapter:** 6

5. Adair 65
- **Meaning:** "oak tree ford"
- **Description:** Of Scottish and Gaelic origin, Adair is a graceful, nature-inspired name signifying strength and tranquility.
- **Chapter:** 3

6. Adrian 24
- **Meaning:** "man of Adria"
- **Description:** Of Latin origin, Adrian evokes sophistication and strength and is associated with Roman emperors and intellectuals.
- **Chapter:** 2

7. Aiden 85
- **Meaning**: "little fire"
- **Description**: Of Irish origin, Aiden is tied to warmth, energy, and vitality, symbolizing spirited strength and determination.
- **Chapter:** 4

8. Alan 18
- **Meaning:** "little rock" or "handsome"

- **Description:** A name of Celtic origin, Alan is a classic, versatile choice symbolizing steadfastness and charm.
- **Chapter:** 2

9. Alden..48
- **Meaning:** "old friend"
- **Description:** A gentle, Old English name symbolizing loyalty, wisdom, and reliability.
- **Chapter:** 3

10. Alexander 24
- **Meaning:** "defender of men" or "protector of humankind"
- **Description:** A strong name associated with Alexander the Great, symbolizing courage, ambition, and leadership.
- **Chapter:** 2

11. Amias..65
- **Meaning:** "beloved"
- **Description:** A Latin and French name symbolizing love, warmth, and compassion.
- **Chapter:** 3

12. Andre..53
- **Meaning:** "manly" or "courageous"
- **Description:** Of Greek origin, Andre is a strong, classic name that signifies bravery and determination, often linked to the variant Andrew.
- **Chapter:** 3

13. Andrew **25**
- **Meaning:** "manly" or "brave"
- **Description:** A Greek-origin name symbolizing strength and courage, associated with the apostle Andrew.
- **Chapter:** 2

14. Angelo **114**
- **Meaning:** "angel" or "messenger"
- **Description:** Of Italian and Greek origin, Angelo represents purity and guidance, often associated with divine inspiration.
- **Chapter:** 6

15. Anthony **18**
- **Meaning:** "priceless one"
- **Description:** Derived from the Roman family name Antonius, this Latin-origin name symbolizes uniqueness and value, with spiritual connections to Saint Anthony of Padua.
- **Chapter:** 2

16. Apollo **85**
- **Meaning:** "god of music, poetry, and healing"
- **Description:** A Greek name symbolizing creativity, light, and truth; associated with the sun.
- **Chapter:** 4

17. Arnold **25**
- **Meaning:** "eagle power"

- **Description:** Of Germanic origin, Arnold symbolizes strength and leadership and is often linked to historic figures of resilience.
- **Chapter:** 2

18. Arthur 25
    - **Meaning:** "bear" or "noble one"
    - **Description:** Inspired by King Arthur, this name carries nobility, bravery, and mystique.
    - **Chapter:** 2

19. Asher 115
    - **Meaning:** "blessed" or "happy"
    - **Description:** A Hebrew name tied to one of Jacob's twelve sons, symbolizing joy and prosperity.
    - **Chapter:** 6

20. Atlas 48
    - **Meaning:** "to carry" or "endure"
    - **Description:** A Greek name inspired by mythology, symbolizing strength and resilience.
    - **Chapter:** 3

21. August 60
    - **Meaning:** "great" or "majestic"
    - **Description:** A Latin name reflecting dignity, leadership, and respect.
    - **Chapter:** 3

22. Aurelio 128
    - **Meaning:** "golden" or "gilded"

- **Description:** A Latin name symbolizing brilliance, warmth, and elegance, derived from the Roman name Aurelius.
- **Chapter:** 6

23. Austin 138
- **Meaning:** "great" or "majestic"
- **Description:** A Latin-derived name connected to the vibrant city of Austin, Texas, known for its creativity and culture.
- **Chapter:** 7

24. Beckett 53
- **Meaning:** "bee cottage"
- **Description:** An Old English surname-turned-first name, Beckett reflects industriousness and charm with a modern twist.
- **Chapter:** 3

25. Benjamin 42
- **Meaning:** "son of the right hand"
- **Description:** A Hebrew name tied to biblical history, symbolizing loyalty and prosperity.
- **Chapter:** 2

26. Benson 49
- **Meaning:** "son of Ben"
- **Description:** Of Old English origin, Benson is a strong and traditional name with familial ties, symbolizing warmth and connection.
- **Chapter:** 3

27. Bodhi 115
- **Meaning:** "awakening" or "enlightenment"
- **Description:** Of Sanskrit origin, Bodhi is tied to spiritual growth and wisdom and is often associated with Buddhist traditions.
- **Chapter:** 6

28. Bruce 26
- **Meaning:** "thick brush" or "willowlands"
- **Description:** Of Scottish and Norman origin, Bruce conveys strength and loyalty and is famously associated with Robert the Bruce of Scotland.
- **Chapter:** 2

29. Bruno 129
- **Meaning:** "brown"
- **Description:** Of Germanic origin, Bruno signifies strength and resilience and is often associated with earthy tones and steadfast character.
- **Chapter:** 6

30. Byron 144
- **Meaning:** "barn for cows"
- **Description:** Associated with poet Lord Byron, this name exudes creativity, romance, and intellectual depth.
- **Chapter:** 7

31. Caelus 86
- **Meaning:** "sky" or "heavens"

- **Description:** A Latin name tied to the Roman god personifying the celestial realm.
- **Chapter:** 4

32. Cairo 144
- **Meaning:** "the strong" or "the victorious"
- **Description:** An Egyptian name reflecting strength and cultural heritage that is tied to the bustling capital city.
- **Chapter:** 7

33. Caleb 122
- **Meaning:** "wholehearted" or "loyal"
- **Description:** A Hebrew name celebrating faith and devotion, with biblical roots tied to Moses's companion.
- **Chapter:** 6

34. Calix 49
- **Meaning:** "very handsome"
- **Description:** A Greek name exuding elegance, charm, and allure.
- **Chapter:** 3

35. Carver 65
- **Meaning:** "woodworker"
- **Description:** Of English origin, Carver symbolizes craftsmanship and creativity, evoking strength and skill.
- **Chapter:** 3

36. Casimir 123

- **Meaning:** "proclaimer of peace"
- **Description:** A Polish name with royal ties, associated with historical leaders who valued wisdom and harmony.
- **Chapter:** 6

37. Cedric..66
- **Meaning:** "kindly and loved"
- **Description:** With Celtic and Old English roots, Cedric carries a noble and gentle quality, perfect for a charismatic individual.
- **Chapter:** 3

38. Charles 19
- **Meaning:** "free man"
- **Description:** Known for historical figures like Charlemagne, Charles represents freedom, responsibility, and integrity.
- **Chapter:** 2

39. Christopher..123
- **Meaning:** "bearing Christ"
- **Description:** A Greek name with spiritual significance that is linked to Saint Christopher, the protector of travelers.
- **Chapter:** 6

40. Cian 129
- **Meaning:** "ancient" or "enduring one"
- **Description:** An Irish name reflecting resilience and rooted in Celtic mythology.
- **Chapter:** 6

41. Clarence 26
- **Meaning**: "bright" or "clear"
- **Description**: Of Latin origin, Clarence has a regal air, historically associated with English nobility.
- **Chapter:** 2

42. Clay 81
- **Meaning**: "mortal" or "clay worker"
- **Description**: Of Old English origin, Clay represents simplicity and strength, symbolizing connection to the earth.
- **Chapter:** 4

43. Colson 66
- **Meaning:** "son of Nicholas"
- **Description:** a modern English surname-inspired name, Colson combines tradition with contemporary style.
- **Chapter:** 3

44. Colton 66
- **Meaning:** "from the coal town"
- **Description:** Of Old English origin, Colton reflects strength and industriousness, offering a rugged and modern vibe.
- **Chapter:** 3

45. Corbin 54
- **Meaning:** "raven"

- **Description:** Of Latin origin, Corbin is associated with mystery and intelligence, offering a name full of depth and charm.
- **Chapter:** 3

46. Cyrus 60
- **Meaning:** "sun" or "lord"
- **Description:** A Persian name linked to wisdom, leadership, and vitality.
- **Chapter:** 3

47. Dalton 49
- **Meaning:** "from the valley town"
- **Description:** An English surname-turned-first name, Dalton is sophisticated yet grounded, symbolizing stability and tradition.
- **Chapter:** 3

48. Damon 86
- **Meaning:** "to tame" or "subdue"
- **Description:** Of Greek origin, Damon reflects loyalty and friendship, inspired by the legendary story of Damon and Pythias.
- **Chapter:** 4

49. Daniel 38
- **Meaning:** "God is my judge"
- **Description:** A Hebrew name associated with faith, wisdom, and resilience.
- **Chapter:** 2

50. Dante 123

- **Meaning:** "steadfast" or "enduring"
- **Description:** A Latin name associated with the author of *The Divine Comedy*, symbolizing spiritual exploration and resilience.
- **Chapter:** 6

51. Darius..66
- **Meaning:** "maintains possessions well"
- **Description:** Of Persian origin, Darius is a regal name tied to ancient kings, symbolizing leadership and strength.
- **Chapter:** 3

52. Dashiell..49
- **Meaning:** "page boy"
- **Description:** A French name with literary connections, Dashiell carries sophistication and a stylish flair.
- **Chapter:** 3

53. Dax...54
- **Meaning:** "leader" or "water"
- **Description:** A bold, modern name with French origins, symbolizing strength and guidance.
- **Chapter:** 3

54. David..32
- **Meaning:** "beloved"
- **Description:** A biblical name with deep historical significance, symbolizing loyalty, strength, and leadership.

- **Chapter:** 2

55. Dean..32
- **Meaning:** "valley"
- **Description:** An English name signifying leadership and humility, Dean balances simplicity with strength.
- **Chapter:** 2

56. Declan..60
- **Meaning:** "man of prayer" or "full of goodness"
- **Description:** An Irish name tied to Saint Declan, symbolizing faith and integrity, with a strong cultural heritage.
- **Chapter:** 3

57. Denver...145
- **Meaning:** "green valley"
- **Description:** A strong name tied to Colorado's vibrant capital, symbolizing adventure and natural beauty.
- **Chapter:** 7

58. Desmond 49
- **Meaning:** "from South Munster"
- **Description:** Of Irish origin, Desmond is a distinguished name tied to heritage and strength, symbolizing wisdom and resilience.
- **Chapter:** 3

59. Dion 67

- **Meaning:** "child of heaven and earth"
- **Description:** Of Greek origin, Dion is associated with Dionysus, the Greek god of wine and festivity, evoking creativity and vitality.
- **Chapter:** 3

60. Dominic 19
- **Meaning:** "belonging to the Lord"
- **Description:** Of Latin origin, Dominic reflects spiritual devotion, with a strong and confident sound.
- **Chapter:** 2

61. Draven..50
- **Meaning:** "hunter"
- **Description:** A modern name with an edgy appeal, Draven symbolizes courage and adventure, offering a unique choice.
- **Chapter:** 3

62. Dublin 139
- **Meaning:** "black pool"
- **Description:** Of Irish origin, Dublin refers to the capital city of Ireland, symbolizing cultural richness and historical depth.
- **Chapter:** 7

63. Edward 42
- **Meaning:** "wealthy guardian"

- **Description:** A noble name linked to kings and historical leaders, symbolizing strength and loyalty.
- **Chapter:** 2

64. Egal 60
- **Meaning:** "equal"
- **Description:** Of Somali origin, Egal reflects fairness and balance, symbolizing harmony and strength.
- **Chapter:** 3

65. Elijah 123
- **Meaning:** "the Lord is my God"
- **Description:** A Hebrew name tied to a powerful biblical prophet known for his faith and miracles.
- **Chapter:** 6

66. Eldon 67
- **Meaning:** "old town"
- **Description:** Of Old English origin, Eldon evokes a sense of heritage and groundedness, symbolizing wisdom and reliability.
- **Chapter:** 3

67. Emil 60
- **Meaning:** "rival" or "eager"
- **Description:** Of Latin origin, Emil is a classic European name reflecting ambition and perseverance, with cultural ties across multiple countries.

- **Chapter:** 3

68. Enoch 67
- **Meaning:** "dedicated"
- **Description:** A biblical name of Hebrew origin, Enoch represents devotion and wisdom, often tied to prophetic insight.
- **Chapter:** 3

69. Ephraim 123
- **Meaning:** "fruitful"
- **Description:** A Hebrew name connected to one of Joseph's sons, symbolizing blessings and growth.
- **Chapter:** 6

70. Ethan 32
- **Meaning:** "strong" or "firm"
- **Description:** A timeless Hebrew name symbolizing endurance and dependability.
- **Chapter:** 2

71. Evander 87
- **Meaning:** "good man" or "strong man"
- **Description:** A Greek name reflecting strength, integrity, and Trojan war heroism.
- **Chapter:** 4

72. Ezra 116
- **Meaning:** "help" or "Yah helps"

- **Description**: Of Hebrew origin, Ezra is tied to wisdom and support, representing resilience and guidance through its biblical roots.
- **Chapter**: 6

73. Finnegan 61
- **Meaning**: "white" or "fair-haired"
- **Description:** An Irish name tied to mythology, bravery, and literary charm.
- **Chapter**: 3

74. Flint..55
- **Meaning**: "hard rock" or "stream"
- **Description**: Of Old English origin, Flint is a strong, rugged name that reflects resilience and natural strength.
- **Chapter**: 3

75. Forrest...82
- **Meaning**: "dweller near the woods"
- **Description**: Of Old French origin, Forrest reflects a love for nature and adventure, embodying resilience and a grounded spirit.
- **Chapter**: 4

76. Frederick..20
- **Meaning**: "peaceful ruler"
- **Description**: Of Germanic origin, Frederick combines strength and serenity, often associated with royalty and scholars.
- **Chapter**: 2

77. Gabriel
- **Meaning:** "man of God"
- **Description:** A Hebrew name of the archangel who appears in both Christian and Islamic traditions, symbolizing strength and divine messages.
- **Chapter:** 6

78. George..........20
- **Meaning:** "farmer" or "earthworker"
- **Description:** A grounded, humble name often associated with English royalty and quiet dignity.
- **Chapter:** 2

79. Gideon..........68
- **Meaning:** "mighty warrior"
- **Description:** Of Hebrew origin, Gideon is a biblical name symbolizing strength and leadership, perfect for a bold and brave individual.
- **Chapter:** 3

80. Graham..........33
- **Meaning:** "gravelly homestead"
- **Description:** Of Scottish origin, Graham is a distinguished and modern-sounding name with traditional roots.
- **Chapter:** 2

81. Gregory..........20
- **Meaning:** "watcher" or "vigilant"

- **Description:** A Greek name of Christian significance, Gregory represents wisdom and vigilance, borne by saints and scholars.
- **Chapter:** 2

82. Griffin..50
- **Meaning:** "lord" or "descendant of the fierce warrior"
- **Description:** A Welsh and Irish name inspired by a mythical creature, symbolizing courage and wisdom.
- **Chapter:** 3

83. Harlan..68
- **Meaning:** "rocky land"
- **Description:** Of English origin, Harlan represents resilience and stability, ideal for a steadfast and dependable personality.
- **Chapter:** 3

84. Harold..43
- **Meaning:** "ruler of the army"
- **Description:** An Old English name symbolizing leadership and tradition.
- **Chapter:** 2

85. Henry..20
- **Meaning:** "house ruler"
- **Description:** A classic royal name embodying strength, simplicity, and warmth.
- **Chapter:** 2

86. Hiroshi 130
- **Meaning:** "tolerant," "generous," or "prosperous"
- **Description:** A Japanese name embodying kindness, grace, and hospitality.
- **Chapter:** 6

87. Holden 55
- **Meaning:** "hollow valley"
- **Description:** Of Old English origin, Holden is a literary name popularized by J.D. Salinger's *The Catcher in the Rye*.
- **Chapter:** 3

88. Homer..55
- **Meaning:** "hostage" or "pledge"
- **Description:** Of Greek origin, Homer honors the legendary poet of *Iliad* and *Odyssey*, symbolizing creativity and storytelling.
- **Chapter:** 3

89. Idris 130
- **Meaning:** "interpreter" or "studious"
- **Description:** Of Arabic and Welsh origin, Idris honors wisdom and learning, associated with a prophet in Islamic tradition and Welsh mythology.
- **Chapter:** 6

90. Ignacio 124
- **Meaning:** "fiery one"

- **Description:** Of Spanish and Latin origin, Ignacio is tied to passion and energy, symbolizing determination and inspiration.
- **Chapter:** 6

91. Ikaros 87
- **Meaning:** "the one who reaches the sky"
- **Description:** A Greek name inspired by the mythological Icarus, symbolizing ambition tempered with wisdom.
- **Chapter:** 4

92. Isaiah 124
- **Meaning:** "salvation of the Lord"
- **Description:** A Hebrew name of a major prophet in the Bible that is associated with hope, redemption, and spiritual insight.
- **Chapter:** 6

93. Ishaan 131
- **Meaning:** "sun" or "lord of wealth"
- **Description:** Of Sanskrit origin, Ishaan symbolizes brightness and prosperity and is often linked to Hindu mythology.
- **Chapter:** 6

94. Ivo 55
- **Meaning:** "yew tree" or "God is gracious"
- **Description:** A German and Hebrew name symbolizing resilience and divine grace.
- **Chapter:** 3

95. Jack **33**
- **Meaning:** "God is gracious"
- **Description:** A British-origin name with charm and vitality that is connected to John and Jacob.
- **Chapter:** 2

96. Jackson **145**
- **Meaning:** "son of Jack"
- **Description:** A timeless name with American roots, Jackson conveys strength, leadership, and approachability.
- **Chapter:** 7

97. Jacob **39**
- **Meaning:** "supplanter"
- **Description:** A Hebrew classic symbolizing determination and adaptability that is rooted in biblical tradition.
- **Chapter:** 2

98. James **20**
- **Meaning:** "supplanter" or "holder of the heel"
- **Description:** A regal name tied to historical leaders and royalty, symbolizing resilience and trustworthiness.
- **Chapter:** 2

99. Jasper **118**
- **Meaning:** "bringer of treasure"
- **Description:** Of Persian origin, Jasper is linked to richness and protection and is historically tied to one of the Three Wise Men.

- **Chapter:** 6

100. Joaquim 118
- **Meaning:** "established by God"
- **Description:** Of Hebrew origin, Joaquim is a biblical name representing faith and strength and is linked to enduring spiritual values.
- **Chapter:** 6

101. Joel 33
- **Meaning:** "Yahweh is God"
- **Description:** A Hebrew name of spiritual depth, Joel is a biblical classic tied to leadership and devotion.
- **Chapter:** 2

102. John 39
- **Meaning:** "God is gracious"
- **Description:** A biblical name known for its simplicity, strength, and universal appeal.
- **Chapter:** 2

103. Joseph 43
- **Meaning:** "God will increase" or "He shall add"
- **Description:** A timeless name with biblical roots, representing loyalty, humility, and resilience.
- **Chapter:** 2

104. Joshua 27
- **Meaning:** "God is salvation"

- **Description:** A Hebrew name of biblical origin, Joshua signifies leadership and faith and is popular across generations.
- **Chapter:** 2

105. Julian 27
- **Meaning:** "youthful" or "downy-bearded"
- **Description:** Of Latin origin, Julian is a refined name with historical and literary connections, symbolizing vitality and intellect.
- **Chapter:** 2

106. Justin 34
- **Meaning:** "just" or "fair"
- **Description:** Of Latin origin, Justin reflects integrity and honor and is often associated with leadership and moral strength.
- **Chapter:** 2

107. Kade 61
- **Meaning:** "round" or "barrel"
- **Description:** Of Scottish origin, Kade is a strong, modern name with simplicity and an adventurous spirit.
- **Chapter:** 3

108. Kavi 69
- **Meaning:** "wise poet"
- **Description:** An Indian name reflecting creativity and intellectual depth.
- **Chapter:** 3

109. Kayden..50
- **Meaning:** "companion" or "fighter"
- **Description:** Of Arabic and Celtic origins, Kayden reflects strength, loyalty, and a modern, spirited energy.
- **Chapter:** 3

110. Keanu...55
- **Meaning:** "cool breeze over the mountains"
- **Description:** Of Hawaiian origin, Keanu evokes serenity and natural beauty and is popularized by actor Keanu Reeves.
- **Chapter:** 3

111. Kendrick 131
- **Meaning:** "royal power" or "champion"
- **Description:** Of English and Scottish origin, Kendrick conveys strength and leadership and is often tied to heritage and resilience.
- **Chapter:** 6

112. Kenzo 61
- **Meaning:** "strong and healthy"
- **Description:** A Japanese name symbolizing vitality and creativity, Kenzo brings a stylish and contemporary appeal.
- **Chapter:** 3

113. Kieran 56
- **Meaning:** "little dark one"
- **Description:** An Irish name combining tradition and modern appeal.

- **Chapter:** 3

114. Kingston..140
- **Meaning:** "king's town"
- **Description:** A regal name tied to the Jamaican capital, symbolizing strength, pride, and a connection to heritage.
- **Chapter:** 7

115. Kwame..131
- **Meaning:** "born on Saturday"
- **Description:** A Ghanaian name from the Akan tradition, reflecting cultural pride and ancestry.
- **Chapter:** 6

116. Lamar 82
- **Meaning:** "the water"
- **Description:** Of Old French origin, Lamar symbolizes fluidity and adaptability, with ties to nature and calm strength.
- **Chapter:** 4

117. Lawrence 28
- **Meaning:** "from Laurentum"
- **Description:** Of Latin origin, Lawrence represents honor and wisdom and is often associated with saints and scholars.
- **Chapter:** 2

118. Leander..88
- **Meaning:** "lion-man"

- **Description:** A Greek name symbolizing courage and loyalty and inspired by mythology.
- **Chapter:** 4

119. Leonardo 132
- **Meaning:** "lion-hearted"
- **Description:** A Germanic-origin name representing courage and strength, with cultural ties to Leonardo da Vinci and the diminutive variant Leo.
- **Chapter:** 6

120. Levent 61
- **Meaning:** "handsome" or "strong"
- **Description:** A Turkish and Greek name associated with nobility and strength.
- **Chapter:** 3

121. Levi 118
- **Meaning:** "joined"
- **Description:** A Hebrew name linked to the Levite tribe, symbolizing unity and spiritual leadership.
- **Chapter:** 6

122. Liam 34
- **Meaning**: "strong-willed warrior"
- **Description**: Of Irish origin, Liam is a short form of William, representing resilience and leadership with contemporary charm.
- **Chapter:** 2

123. Loki 88
- **Meaning:** "lock"
- **Description:** A Norse name associated with the god of mischief, symbolizing adaptability and reinvention.
- **Chapter:** 4

124. Louis 28
- **Meaning:** "renowned warrior"
- **Description:** A regal name carried by French royalty, symbolizing strength and grandeur.
- **Chapter:** 2

125. Lucien 69
- **Meaning:** "light"
- **Description:** Of French and Latin origin, Lucien is associated with enlightenment and clarity, symbolizing creativity and intellect.
- **Chapter:** 3

126. Luke 34
- **Meaning:** "light-giving"
- **Description:** A Greek name symbolizing wisdom, kindness, and illumination.
- **Chapter:** 2

127. Malachi 132
- **Meaning:** "messenger of God"
- **Description:** A Hebrew name from the Bible, representing spiritual depth and the role of a divine communicator.
- **Chapter:** 6

128. Malcolm...61
- **Meaning:** "devotee of Saint Columba"
- **Description:** Of Scottish origin, Malcolm reflects heritage and dignity and is often associated with leadership and intellect.
- **Chapter:** 3

129. Malik..132
- **Meaning:** "king" or "ruler"
- **Description:** Of Arabic origin, Malik embodies leadership and strength, reflecting dignity and authority.
- **Chapter:** 6

130. Marcelo...132
- **Meaning:** "little warrior"
- **Description:** Of Italian and Latin origin, Marcelo reflects courage and vitality and is often linked to cultural refinement and strength.
- **Chapter:** 6

131. Mark..35
- **Meaning:** "war-like" or "dedicated to Mars"
- **Description:** A name with biblical and Roman significance, representing strength and quiet confidence.
- **Chapter:** 2

132. Marshall..40
- **Meaning:** "horse caretaker" or "steward"

- **Description:** Of Old French origin, Marshall signifies responsibility and leadership and is often associated with loyalty and honor.
- **Chapter:** 2

133. Martin 124
- **Meaning:** "of Mars" or "war-like"
- **Description:** Of Latin origin, Martin is tied to the Roman god of war, symbolizing courage and strategy.
- **Chapter:** 6

134. Mason 21
- **Meaning:** "stoneworker"
- **Description:** An English occupational name symbolizing craftsmanship, strength, and reliability.
- **Chapter:** 2

135. Mateo 124
- **Meaning:** "gift of God"
- **Description:** A Spanish variation of Matthew, reflecting gratitude and faith, that is widely used across cultures.
- **Chapter:** 6

136. Matthew 118
- **Meaning:** "gift of God"
- **Description:** A Hebrew name associated with Saint Matthew, one of the Twelve Apostles, symbolizing gratitude and faith.
- **Chapter:** 6

137. Michael 119
- **Meaning:** "who resembles God?"
- **Description:** A Hebrew name of the archangel leading heaven's armies, symbolizing protection and strength.
- **Chapter:** 6

138. Miles 28
- **Meaning:** "merciful" or "soldier"
- **Description:** A Latin and Germanic name with historical and modern heroism.
- **Chapter:** 2

139. Mohammed 125
- **Meaning:** "praiseworthy" or "commendable"
- **Description:** An Arabic name of great spiritual significance as the name of Prophet Muhammad, symbolizing high moral qualities.
- **Chapter:** 6

140. Moses 119
- **Meaning:** "drawn out"
- **Description:** Of Hebrew origin, Moses is a biblical name associated with leadership and deliverance, reflecting spiritual guidance and strength.
- **Chapter:** 6

141. Nathaniel...119
- **Meaning:** "God has given"

- **Description:** A Hebrew name symbolizing faith and gratitude, mentioned in both the Old and New Testament.
- **Chapter:** 6

142. Neil..35
- **Meaning:** "champion" or "cloud"
- **Description:** A name of Irish origin, Neil conveys strength and resilience and is celebrated for its simplicity and charm.
- **Chapter:** 2

143. Niall..62
- **Meaning:** "champion"
- **Description:** An Irish name with strong historical ties, Niall symbolizes valor and leadership, blending tradition with a modern edge.
- **Chapter:** 3

144. Nicholas..125
- **Meaning:** "victory of the people"
- **Description:** Of Greek origin, Nicholas represents strength and triumph and is tied to Saint Nicholas and timeless traditions of generosity.
- **Chapter:** 6

145. Nilo 62
- **Meaning:** "Nile River"
- **Description:** A Spanish and Egyptian name representing life, prosperity, and natural beauty.

- **Chapter:** 3

146. Noah **119**
- **Meaning:** "rest" or "motion"
- **Description:** A Hebrew name of the biblical figure who built the Ark, symbolizing resilience and faith.
- **Chapter:** 6

147. Noel..**62**
- **Meaning:** "Christmas" or "born on Christmas"
- **Description:** A French and Latin name embodying warmth, joy, and festivity.
- **Chapter:** 3

148. Oberon...**51**
- **Meaning:** "noble bear" or "king of the fairies"
- **Description:** A Germanic name associated with strength, nobility, and enchantment.
- **Chapter:** 3

149. Odin **89**
- **Meaning:** "frenzy" or "divine inspiration"
- **Description:** A Norse name tied to wisdom, war, and magic from the all-father god of mythology.
- **Chapter:** 4

150. Oliver..**78**
- **Meaning:** "olive tree"
- **Description:** A Latin-origin name symbolizing peace, dignity, and friendship.

- **Chapter:** 4

151. Omar 125
- **Meaning:** "flourishing" or "long-lived"
- **Description:** Of Arabic origin, Omar is a strong and timeless name tied to historical leaders and cultural depth.
- **Chapter:** 6

152. Orion 89
- **Meaning:** "hunter"
- **Description:** A Greek name tied to mythology and the stars, symbolizing adventure and curiosity.
- **Chapter:** 4

153. Orlando 146
- **Meaning:** "glorious land"
- **Description:** Rooted in Italian origins, Orlando carries literary charm from Shakespeare's *As You Like It* as well as a sense of cultural richness.
- **Chapter:** 7

154. Orson 51
- **Meaning:** "bear cub"
- **Description:** Of Latin origin, Orson is bold and endearing, reflecting strength and a connection to nature.
- **Chapter:** 3

155. Oscar 29

- **Meaning:** "God's spear"
- **Description:** Of Irish and Norse origin, Oscar is a bold and heroic name with literary and artistic significance.
- **Chapter:** 2

156. Otis 56
- **Meaning:** "wealth" or "prosperity"
- **Description:** A vintage German name with a charming and approachable feel.
- **Chapter:** 3

157. Otto 63
- **Meaning:** "wealth" or "prosperity"
- **Description:** A German name reflecting abundance and timeless charm.
- **Chapter:** 3

158. Owen 35
- **Meaning:** "young warrior" or "well-born"
- **Description:** Of Welsh origin, Owen reflects strength and valor, with ties to historical and literary figures.
- **Chapter:** 2

159. Patrick 29
- **Meaning:** "nobleman"
- **Description:** Of Latin origin, Patrick is associated with Saint Patrick, the patron saint of Ireland, symbolizing strength and humility.
- **Chapter:** 2

160. Paul 36
- **Meaning:** "small" or "humble"
- **Description:** A Latin name representing modesty and strength, with biblical roots.
- **Chapter:** 2

161. Pax 63
- **Meaning:** "peace"
- **Description:** A Latin name symbolizing harmony and goodwill that is associated with Roman mythology.
- **Chapter:** 3

162. Porter 57
- **Meaning:** "gatekeeper"
- **Description:** Of Old French origin, Porter symbolizes responsibility and hospitality, offering a name full of charm and purpose.
- **Chapter:** 3

163. Quentin 51
- **Meaning:** "fifth"
- **Description:** Of Latin origin, Quentin is traditionally used for a fifth-born child, symbolizing uniqueness and historical depth.
- **Chapter:** 3

164. Rafael 119
- **Meaning:** "God has healed"
- **Description:** Of Hebrew origin, Rafael conveys spiritual renewal and protection and is often associated with the archangel in biblical texts.

- **Chapter:** 6

165. Rafferty 70
- **Meaning:** "prosperity wielder" or "flood tide"
- **Description:** An Irish name with rhythmic energy and charm.
- **Chapter:** 3

166. Rami 133
- **Meaning:** "archer"
- **Description:** An Arabic and Hebrew name symbolizing focus and determination and associated with precision and strength.
- **Chapter:** 6

167. Ravi 133
- **Meaning:** "sun"
- **Description:** Of Sanskrit origin, Ravi symbolizes light, energy, and vitality, celebrated as a divine force in Hindu traditions.
- **Chapter:** 6

168. Reed 78
- **Meaning:** "red-haired" or "reed plant"
- **Description:** Of Old English origin, Reed symbolizes adaptability and harmony and is often tied to nature and musicality.
- **Chapter:** 4

169. Richard 22
- **Meaning:** "brave ruler"

- **Description:** Of Germanic origin, Richard is a classic name associated with kings and leaders, symbolizing courage and power.
- **Chapter:** 2

170. River 83
- **Meaning:** "flowing body of water"
- **Description:** A serene and adaptable name reflecting life's journey and natural beauty.
- **Chapter:** 4

171. Robert 23
- **Meaning:** "bright fame"
- **Description:** Of Germanic origin, Robert is a timeless and noble name with historical and familial significance.
- **Chapter:** 2

172. Rohan 133
- **Meaning:** "ascending"
- **Description:** Of Sanskrit origin, Rohan represents growth and ambition and is also popular in Irish traditions, meaning "red-haired."
- **Chapter:** 6

173. Roman 63
- **Meaning:** "citizen of Rome"
- **Description:** Of Latin origin, Roman evokes strength, history, and a connection to the grandeur of the Roman Empire.
- **Chapter:** 3

174. Ronan **141**
- **Meaning:** "little seal"
- **Description:** An Irish name with connections to the sea and Celtic mythology, embodying resilience and humor.
- **Chapter:** 7

175. Ross **57**
- **Meaning:** "promontory" or "headland"
- **Description:** Of Scottish and Gaelic origin, Ross connects to natural landscapes and heritage, symbolizing strength and stability.
- **Chapter:** 3

176. Ryder **51**
- **Meaning:** "cavalryman" or "messenger"
- **Description:** Of Old English origin, Ryder is a bold, modern name symbolizing movement and determination.
- **Chapter:** 3

177. Ryker **52**
- **Meaning**: "powerful" or "rich"
- **Description**: Of Dutch origin, Ryker conveys fortitude and prosperity, often linked to a bold and modern identity.
- **Chapter:** 3

178. Samuel **44**
- **Meaning:** "God has heard"

- **Description:** A biblical name symbolizing wisdom, resilience, and spirituality.
- **Chapter:** 2

179. Santiago 125
- **Meaning:** "Saint James"
- **Description:** A Spanish name honoring Saint James the Great, symbolizing strength and devotion.
- **Chapter:** 6

180. Sebastian 126
- **Meaning:** "venerable" or "revered"
- **Description:** A Latin name with associations of elegance, strength, and resilience.
- **Chapter:** 6

181. Seraphim 120
- **Meaning:** "the burning one"
- **Description:** A Hebrew name referring to the highest-ranking angels, symbolizing divine strength and passion.
- **Chapter:** 6

182. Seth 36
- **Meaning:** "appointed" or "placed"
- **Description:** A Hebrew name of biblical origin, Seth represents strength and renewal and is often chosen for its simplicity.
- **Chapter:** 2

183. Simon 126

- **Meaning:** "to hear" or "listening"
- **Description:** A Hebrew and Greek name associated with faith and thoughtfulness and tied to Simon Peter from the Bible.
- **Chapter:** 6

184. Solomon 126
- **Meaning:** "peace"
- **Description:** A Hebrew name of the wise and just biblical king, symbolizing harmony and intellect.
- **Chapter:** 6

185. Soren 57
- **Meaning:** "stern" or "strict"
- **Description:** A Scandinavian name tied to strength, depth, and intellectual legacy.
- **Chapter:** 3

186. Stephen 23
- **Meaning:** "crown"
- **Description:** Of Greek origin, Stephen is a classic and dignified name, symbolizing honor and perseverance.
- **Chapter:** 2

187. Sylvan 79
- **Meaning:** "of the forest"
- **Description:** A Latin name evoking harmony, wisdom, and freedom, inspired by the Roman god of forests.
- **Chapter:** 4

188. Tariq **134**
- **Meaning:** "visitor" or "morning star"
- **Description:** An Arabic name symbolizing arrival, light, and celestial beauty.
- **Chapter:** 6

189. Theodore **30**
- **Meaning:** "gift of God"
- **Description:** A dignified name tied to leadership and wisdom, popularized by President Theodore Roosevelt.
- **Chapter:** 2

190. Thomas **23**
- **Meaning:** "twin"
- **Description:** A steadfast biblical name associated with loyalty, humility, and inventiveness.
- **Chapter:** 2

191. Timothy **126**
- **Meaning:** "honoring God"
- **Description:** Of Greek origin, Timothy reflects devotion and faith, with strong biblical connections to Saint Timothy.
- **Chapter:** 6

192. Tobin **57**
- **Meaning:** "God is good"

- **Description**: Of Hebrew origin, Tobin is a variation of Tobias, reflecting spiritual gratitude and kindness.
- **Chapter**: 3

193. Tristan 70
- **Meaning:** "tumult" or "sorrowful"
- **Description:** Of Celtic origin, Tristan is tied to the legend of Tristan and Isolde, symbolizing romance and bravery.
- **Chapter**: 3

194. Troy 36
- **Meaning:** "foot soldier" or "of Troy"
- **Description:** Of Greek and Irish origin, Troy evokes strength and bravery, tied to the legendary city of Troy.
- **Chapter**: 2

195. Valentino..127
- **Meaning:** "strong" or "healthy"
- **Description:** Of Latin origin, Valentino embodies vitality and resilience and is often associated with elegance and romance.
- **Chapter**: 6

196. Victor 23
- **Meaning:** "conqueror" or "winner"
- **Description:** Of Latin origin, Victor represents triumph and resilience, celebrated through its historical and cultural significance.
- **Chapter**: 2

197. Vincent 30
- **Meaning:** "conquering"
- **Description:** Of Latin origin, Vincent symbolizes determination and success and is famously associated with artist Vincent van Gogh.
- **Chapter:** 2

198. Vlad 57
- **Meaning:** "ruler" or "prince"
- **Description:** Of Slavic origin, Vlad is a strong, commanding name tied to history and legend, including Vlad the Impaler.
- **Chapter:** 3

199. Wallace 44
- **Meaning:** "foreigner"
- **Description:** Of Old French and Scottish origin, Wallace is tied to history and strength, famously linked to the Scottish hero William Wallace.
- **Chapter:** 2

200. William..23
- **Meaning:** "resolute protector" or "strong-willed warrior"
- **Description:** A name of historical significance, symbolizing strength and adaptability.
- **Chapter:** 2

201. Xander 52

- **Meaning**: "defender of the people"
- **Description**: Of Greek origin, Xander is a modern short form of Alexander, embodying courage and leadership.
- **Chapter:** 3

202. Zachary 121
- **Meaning:** "the Lord recalled"
- **Description:** A Hebrew name tied to biblical roots, offering nicknames like Zach or Zack.
- **Chapter:** 6

203. Zane 71
- **Meaning:** "God is gracious"
- **Description:** A Hebrew name with a modern feel, Zane exudes simplicity and strength, offering a bold and fresh choice.
- **Chapter:** 3

204. Zurich 151
- **Meaning:** "belonging to Tūros"
- **Description:** A Latin-derived name reflecting Switzerland's largest city, known for its sophistication and cultural depth.
- **Chapter:** 7

Girl Names

1. Abigail 31
- **Meaning:** "my father's joy"

- **Description:** A name symbolizing wisdom, eloquence, and beauty that is rooted in biblical tradition.
- **Chapter:** 2

2. Acacia 65
- **Meaning:** "thorny tree" or "resurrection"
- **Description:** Of Greek origin, Acacia symbolizes resilience and immortality, which are often associated with the Acacia tree's enduring nature.
- **Chapter:** 3

3. Adriana..37
- **Meaning:** "from Hadria"
- **Description:** Of Latin origin, Adriana reflects refinement and cultural depth and is tied to elegance and strength.
- **Chapter:** 2

4. Aisha..122
- **Meaning:** "alive and well"
- **Description:** An Arabic name honoring Prophet Muhammad's wife, symbolizing resilience and charm.
- **Chapter:** 6

5. Alexandra 25
- **Meaning:** "defender of mankind"
- **Description:** Of Greek origin, Alexandra is a timeless and elegant name associated with

royalty and strength, often shortened to Alex, Lexi, or Sandy.
- **Chapter:** 2

6. Alice 31
- **Meaning:** "noble" or "exalted"
- **Description:** A classic, elegant name tied to curiosity and adventure, popularized by *Alice in Wonderland*.
- **Chapter:** 2

7. Alissa..59
- **Meaning:** "nobility" or "wanderer"
- **Description:** A name with German and Arabic roots, symbolizing grace, dignity, curiosity, and exploration, with flexible variations like Alyssa and Elissa.
- **Chapter:** 3

8. Alora..48
- **Meaning:** "my dream"
- **Description:** A Bantu and Latin name symbolizing aspiration, beauty, and growth.
- **Chapter:** 3

9. Amani 128
- **Meaning:** "peace" or "wishes"
- **Description:** An Arabic and Swahili name that conveys a sense of hope and serenity, often chosen for its uplifting significance.
- **Chapter:** 6

10. Amara 59
- **Meaning:** "everlasting" or "grace"
- **Description:** A multicultural name signifying love, vitality, and the enduring spirit.
- **Chapter:** 3

11. Amelia 41
- **Meaning:** "industrious" or "striving"
- **Description:** A Latin name emphasizing ambition and integrity.
- **Chapter:** 2

12. Amelie 37
- **Meaning:** "hardworking"
- **Description:** A French variation of Amelia, Amelie evokes charm, creativity, and diligence, with literary and cinematic ties.
- **Chapter:** 2

13. Amina 128
- **Meaning:** "safe one" or "faithful"
- **Description:** An Arabic name embodying trustworthiness and integrity.
- **Chapter:** 6

14. Ananya 59
- **Meaning:** "unique" or "incomparable"
- **Description:** Of Sanskrit origin, Ananya reflects singularity and grace, embodying qualities of distinction and elegance.
- **Chapter:** 3

15. Anjali..128
- **Meaning:** "divine offering"
- **Description:** A Sanskrit name reflecting reverence, grace, and cultural connection.
- **Chapter:** 6

16. Anna 37
- **Meaning:** "grace" or "favor"
- **Description:** A simple, elegant Hebrew name symbolizing kindness and resilience.
- **Chapter:** 2

17. Annabelle...42
- **Meaning:** "lovable"
- **Description:** A French-origin name blending Anna and Belle, it symbolizes grace and beauty with a lyrical quality.
- **Chapter:** 2

18. Anya..38
- **Meaning:** "grace"
- **Description:** Of Russian and Hebrew origins, Anya is a simple yet elegant name reflecting kindness and charm.
- **Chapter:** 2

19. Arabella 38
- **Meaning:** "yielding to prayer"
- **Description:** A Latin-origin name exuding refinement, it carries a regal, romantic quality tied to history and literature.
- **Chapter:** 2

20. Ariana **128**
- **Meaning:** "most holy" or "silver"
- **Description:** Derived from Greek and Welsh origins, this name reflects purity, sacredness, and rarity.
- **Chapter:** 6

21. Arlette **65**
- **Meaning:** "lion of God"
- **Description:** A French name with Hebrew roots, Arlette combines elegance with strength, making it a timeless and unique choice.
- **Chapter:** 3

22. Artemis **85**
- **Meaning:** "twin of Apollo"
- **Description:** A Greek name referring to the goddess of the moon, hunting, and wilderness, embodying strength and freedom.
- **Chapter:** 4

23. Arwen **59**
- **Meaning:** "noble maiden" or "muse"
- **Description:** A Welsh name reflecting grace, bravery, and literary charm.
- **Chapter:** 3

24. Astrid **59**
- **Meaning:** "divinely beautiful"

- **Description:** Of Scandinavian origin, Astrid was historically used by Nordic royalty and exudes grace and nobility.
- **Chapter:** 3

25. Athena 85
- **Meaning:** "goddess of wisdom and war"
- **Description:** A Greek name symbolizing intelligence, strategy, and protection.
- **Chapter:** 4

26. Audrey 122
- **Meaning:** "noble strength"
- **Description:** Of Old English origin, this classic name is known for its association with Audrey Hepburn, symbolizing grace and sophistication.
- **Chapter:** 6

27. Aura 81
- **Meaning:** "gentle breeze" or "air"
- **Description:** A Latin and Greek name reflecting calm, clarity, and ethereal beauty.
- **Chapter:** 4

28. Aurora 85
- **Meaning:** "dawn"
- **Description:** A Latin name symbolizing new beginnings and light, associated with the Roman goddess of sunrise.
- **Chapter:** 4

29. Autumn 81
- **Meaning:** "season of harvest"
- **Description:** A Latin name representing transformation, reflection, and abundance.
- **Chapter:** 4

30. Ava 129
- **Meaning:** "bird," "life," or "voice"
- **Description:** A Latin, Hebrew, and Persian name evoking grace, vitality, and lyrical energy.
- **Chapter:** 6

31. Avalon 147
- **Meaning:** "island of apples"
- **Description:** A mythical name tied to Arthurian legend, Avalon represents mystique, serenity, and an idyllic paradise.
- **Chapter:** 7

32. Azalea 74
- **Meaning:** "dry"
- **Description:** A Greek name inspired by the vibrant flowering shrub, reflecting resilience and beauty.
- **Chapter:** 4

33. Azura 49
- **Meaning:** "sky blue"
- **Description:** A serene name with Persian roots, evoking natural beauty and calm.
- **Chapter:** 3

34. Beatrice 25
- **Meaning:** "voyager" or "blessed"
- **Description:** A timeless name representing joy, wisdom, and resilience, famously featured in Dante's *Divine Comedy*.
- **Chapter:** 2

35. Brianna 129
- **Meaning:** "noble" or "high"
- **Description:** An Irish-origin name that combines strength and femininity, Brianna symbolizes dignity and resilience.
- **Chapter:** 6

36. Brielle 60
- **Meaning:** "God is my strength"
- **Description:** Of French and Hebrew origin, Brielle is a modern and graceful name, often seen as a shortened form of Gabrielle.
- **Chapter:** 3

37. Brigid 122
- **Meaning:** "exalted one"
- **Description:** Of Irish origin, Brigid is tied to the Celtic goddess of poetry, fire, and healing as well as Saint Brigid, a revered Irish figure.
- **Chapter:** 6

38. Brittany...31
- **Meaning:** "from Britain"

- **Description:** Derived from the French region of Bretagne, Brittany became popular in the late 20th century, evoking charm and vitality.
- **Chapter:** 2

39. Brynn..53
- **Meaning:** "hill"
- **Description:** Of Welsh origin, Brynn is a sleek and modern name evoking natural beauty and simplicity.
- **Chapter:** 3

40. Calista 86
- **Meaning:** "most beautiful"
- **Description:** A Greek name symbolizing grace and celestial beauty, Calista is tied to mythology.
- **Chapter:** 4

41. Calliope 86
- **Meaning:** "beautiful voice"
- **Description:** A Greek name inspired by the muse of epic poetry, symbolizing creativity and eloquence.
- **Chapter:** 4

42. Camila..115
- **Meaning:** "religious attendant"
- **Description:** A Latin name symbolizing devotion and cultural depth and tied to

Roman history, with diminutives like Milla or Millie.
- **Chapter:** 6

43. Carmen..38
- **Meaning:** "song" or "poem"
- **Description:** Of Latin origin, Carmen carries cultural richness and is widely associated with the famous opera by Bizet.
- **Chapter:** 2

44. Caroline..42
- **Meaning:** "free woman"
- **Description:** A Germanic name blending sophistication, independence, and warmth.
- **Chapter:** 2

45. Cassia 54
- **Meaning:** "cinnamon"
- **Description:** A Greek name linked to the fragrant spice, Cassia evokes warmth and sweetness while maintaining a modern edge.
- **Chapter:** 3

46. Cassidy 65
- **Meaning:** "clever" or "curly-haired"
- **Description:** An Irish-origin name, Cassidy is lively and friendly, often associated with creativity and charm.
- **Chapter:** 3

47. Catherine...26

- **Meaning:** "pure"
- **Description:** A royal and virtuous name carried by queens and saints, symbolizing elegance and strength.
- **Chapter:** 2

48. Cecilia 26
- **Meaning:** "blind"
- **Description:** A Latin name with rich historical roots and often associated with Saint Cecilia, the patroness of music.
- **Chapter:** 2

49. Charity 115
- **Meaning:** "giving" or "kindness"
- **Description:** A British virtue name emphasizing generosity and selflessness, popular since the Puritan era.
- **Chapter:** 6

50. Charlotte...................19
- **Meaning:** "free man"
- **Description:** A sophisticated and historic name linked to royalty, blending strength and femininity.
- **Chapter:** 2

51. Cheyenne 144
- **Meaning:** "people of a different language"
- **Description:** Of Native American origin, Cheyenne honors the indigenous tribe and symbolizes connection and cultural heritage.

- **Chapter:** 7

52. Chloe 86
- **Meaning:** "young green shoot"
- **Description:** A Greek name linked to fertility, growth, and Demeter, the goddess of agriculture.
- **Chapter:** 4

53. Claire 31
- **Meaning:** "bright" or "clear"
- **Description:** A French name reflecting purity, light, and elegance.
- **Chapter:** 2

54. Clara 32
- **Meaning:** "bright" or "famous"
- **Description:** A Latin name radiating vintage charm and sophistication.
- **Chapter:** 2

55. Cleo 54
- **Meaning:** "glory" or "pride"
- **Description:** A Greek name with regal history and vibrant energy.
- **Chapter:** 3

56. Clover 66
- **Meaning:** "meadow flower"
- **Description:** An English botanical name symbolizing luck and prosperity, Clover brings a fresh and cheerful charm.

- **Chapter:** 3

57. Coral..75
- **Meaning:** "limestone skeleton" or "small stone"
- **Description:** A Latin and Greek name inspired by ocean life, symbolizing resilience and natural beauty.
- **Chapter:** 4

58. Dahlia...75
- **Meaning:** "valley" or "flower"
- **Description:** Of Scandinavian origin, Dahlia is also tied to the elegant and vibrant flower, symbolizing inner strength and beauty.
- **Chapter:** 4

59. Daisy 75
- **Meaning:** "day's eye"
- **Description:** Of Old English origin, Daisy represents innocence and purity, inspired by the cheerful flower that opens with the sun.
- **Chapter:** 4

60. Daphne...86
- **Meaning:** "laurel tree"
- **Description:** Of Greek origin, Daphne is tied to Greek mythology, symbolizing victory and resilience through its connection to the laurel tree.
- **Chapter:** 4

61. Dawn 76
- **Meaning:** "first light of day"
- **Description:** A poetic name representing new beginnings and endless possibilities.
- **Chapter:** 4

62. Daya 66
- **Meaning:** "compassion"
- **Description:** With Sanskrit roots, Daya conveys kindness and empathy, embodying inner peace and grace.
- **Chapter:** 3

63. Delaney 67
- **Meaning:** "from the alder grove"
- **Description:** Of Irish origin, Delaney is a stylish and upbeat name reflecting a connection to nature and heritage.
- **Chapter:** 3

64. Delilah 116
- **Meaning:** "delicate" or "to flirt"
- **Description:** A Hebrew name connected to the biblical figure known for her beauty and complexity, symbolizing strength and allure.
- **Chapter:** 6

65. Delphi 148
- **Meaning:** "womb" or "oracle"
- **Description:** Inspired by the ancient Greek city known for its Oracle, Delphi

symbolizes wisdom, mystery, and spiritual insight.
- **Chapter:** 7

66. Diana..26
- **Meaning:** "divine" or "heavenly"
- **Description:** A name rooted in Roman mythology, symbolizing independence, grace, and protection.
- **Chapter:** 2

67. Ebele..129
- **Meaning:** "mercy" or "kindness"
- **Description:** Of Igbo origin, Ebele reflects compassion and a gentle spirit, celebrating qualities of empathy and grace.
- **Chapter:** 6

68. Eirene...87
- **Meaning**: "peace"
- **Description**: Of Greek origin, Eirene is associated with the goddess of peace in Greek mythology, symbolizing harmony and renewal.
- **Chapter**: 4

69. Elara..87
- **Meaning:** "hazelnut" or "spear shaft"
- **Description:** A Greek name tied to mythology and celestial resonance as one of Jupiter's moons.
- **Chapter:** 4

70. Eleanor..26
- **Meaning:** "shining light" or "bright one"
- **Description:** A regal and intellectual name tied to strong historical figures like Eleanor Roosevelt.
- **Chapter:** 2

71. Eliana...116
- **Meaning:** "God has answered"
- **Description:** A Hebrew name symbolizing faith and gratitude, also connected to the Latin meaning of "sun."
- **Chapter:** 6

72. Elise..32
- **Meaning:** "pledged to God"
- **Description:** A French diminutive of Elizabeth, Elise combines simplicity with spiritual depth and grace.
- **Chapter:** 2

73. Elizabeth..19
- **Meaning:** "God is my oath"
- **Description:** A regal, versatile name cherished for its grace, strength, and universal appeal.
- **Chapter:** 2

74. Ella...42
- **Meaning:** "fairy maiden" or "goddess"

- **Description:** A German-origin name reflecting grace and cultural richness.
- **Chapter:** 2

75. Eloise 129
- **Meaning:** "healthy" or "wide"
- **Description:** Of French and German origin, this name is elegant and classic and often tied to literary and historical significance.
- **Chapter:** 6

76. Elowen 76
- **Meaning:** "elm tree"
- **Description:** A Cornish name symbolizing growth, stability, and grace.
- **Chapter:** 4

77. Emberly 67
- **Meaning:** "burning meadow"
- **Description:** A modern variation of Ember, this name symbolizes warmth and light, perfect for a glowing personality.
- **Chapter:** 3

78. Emily 19
- **Meaning:** "rival" or "laborious"
- **Description:** A Latin-origin name symbolizing perseverance and ambition.
- **Chapter:** 2

79. Emma 19
- **Meaning:** "whole" or "universal"

- **Description:** A warm and elegant name symbolizing kindness and sophistication, popular across generations.
- **Chapter:** 2

80. Esme 54
- **Meaning:** "esteemed" or "loved"
- **Description:** A French name celebrating beauty and value with a gem-like quality.
- **Chapter:** 3

81. Esther..123
- **Meaning:** "star"
- **Description:** A Persian name representing courage and wisdom, tied to the heroine of the Hebrew Bible.
- **Chapter:** 6

82. Evangeline 43
- **Meaning:** "bearer of good news"
- **Description:** A Greek-origin name linked to the gospel, Evangeline evokes inspiration, hope, and lyrical beauty.
- **Chapter:** 2

83. Eve 116
- **Meaning:** "life" or "living being"
- **Description:** A Hebrew name honoring the first woman in the Bible, symbolizing creation and vitality.
- **Chapter:** 6

84. Evie **68**
- **Meaning:** "life"
- **Description:** A Hebrew name symbolizing vitality and new beginnings.
- **Chapter:** 3

85. Faith **117**
- **Meaning:** "trust" or "devotion"
- **Description:** An English virtue name reflecting belief, loyalty, and steadfastness.
- **Chapter:** 6

86. Farah **130**
- **Meaning:** "joy" or "happiness"
- **Description:** Of Arabic origin, Farah conveys a sense of celebration and positivity, embodying light and cheerfulness.
- **Chapter:** 6

87. Faye **55**
- **Meaning:** "fairy" or "belief"
- **Description:** A delicate name with English, French, and Latin origins, evoking trust and magic.
- **Chapter:** 3

88. Fern **76**
- **Meaning:** "shade-loving plant"
- **Description:** An Old English name reflecting humility, resilience, and timeless elegance.
- **Chapter:** 4

89. Fiona **27**
- **Meaning:** "fair" or "white"
- **Description:** Of Scottish and Gaelic origin, Fiona embodies beauty and elegance, with literary ties and a timeless charm.
- **Chapter:** 2

90. Flora **82**
- **Meaning:** "flower"
- **Description:** A Latin name inspired by the Roman goddess of flowers and spring, symbolizing beauty and renewal.
- **Chapter:** 4

91. Florence **139**
- **Meaning:** "blossoming" or "flourishing"
- **Description:** A Latin name celebrating growth and prosperity, linked to the Italian Renaissance city.
- **Chapter:** 7

92. Freya **87**
- **Meaning:** "noble lady"
- **Description:** A Norse name representing beauty, bravery, and fertility.
- **Chapter:** 4

93. Gaia **82**
- **Meaning:** "earth"
- **Description:** A Greek name symbolizing life, growth, and nurturing, drawn from mythology.

- **Chapter:** 4

94. Galadriel 68
- **Meaning:** "maiden crowned with a radiant garland"
- **Description:** A Tolkien-inspired name with ethereal qualities and literary charm.
- **Chapter:** 3

95. Geneva 139
- **Meaning:** "juniper tree" or "bending river"
- **Description:** A German-origin name associated with Switzerland's elegance and neutrality, rich in natural symbolism.
- **Chapter:** 7

96. Genevieve 27
- **Meaning:** "woman," "family," or "white fay"
- **Description:** A French name honoring Saint Genevieve, it blends historical depth with soft, melodic grace.
- **Chapter:** 2

97. Giselle 38
- **Meaning:** "pledge" or "hostage"
- **Description:** Of French and German origin, Giselle carries an elegant, graceful quality, famously tied to the romantic ballet *Giselle*.
- **Chapter:** 2

98. Grace 32
- **Meaning:** "favor" or "blessing"

- **Description:** A Latin name representing divine virtue, elegance, and simplicity.
- **Chapter:** 2

99. Hana 130
- **Meaning:** "happiness" or "flower"
- **Description:** A name with diverse origins (means "flower" in Japanese), embodying joy and beauty, often seen as a variation of Hannah.
- **Chapter:** 6

100. Hania 68
- **Meaning:** "grace" or "happiness"
- **Description:** Of Hebrew and Native American origins, Hania is a sweet and uplifting name symbolizing joy and favor.
- **Chapter:** 3

101. Hannah 117
- **Meaning:** "grace" or "favor"
- **Description:** A Hebrew name from the Bible, Hannah is associated with a woman of faith and prayer, symbolizing divine blessings.
- **Chapter:** 6

102. Harriet 33
- **Meaning:** "ruler of the home"
- **Description:** An Old English name embodying strength and independence, famously borne by Harriet Tubman.
- **Chapter:** 2

103. Hazel 82
- **Meaning:** "hazel tree"
- **Description:** An Old English name symbolizing wisdom, protection, and natural beauty.
- **Chapter:** 4

104. Helen 27
- **Meaning:** "torch" or "light"
- **Description:** A Greek name symbolizing beauty, grace, and strength.
- **Chapter:** 2

105. Holland 148
- **Meaning:** "wooded land"
- **Description:** A Dutch-inspired name evoking scenic beauty and cultural heritage, perfect for those drawn to nature and European charm.
- **Chapter:** 7

106. Hope....................................117
- **Meaning:** "to cherish a desire with anticipation"
- **Description:** A British name symbolizing optimism, resilience, and faith in better days.
- **Chapter:** 6

107. Imara 69
- **Meaning:** "strong" or "steadfast"

- **Description:** A Swahili name reflecting courage and resilience.
- **Chapter:** 3

108. India 139
- **Meaning:** "from the Indus River"
- **Description:** A name of Latin and Sanskrit origins, inspired by the geographic and cultural beauty of South Asia.
- **Chapter:** 7

109. Indira 130
- **Meaning:** "beauty" or "splendor"
- **Description:** A Sanskrit name associated with the goddess Lakshmi, symbolizing prosperity and elegance.
- **Chapter:** 6

110. Inez 131
- **Meaning:** "pure"
- **Description:** A Portuguese and Spanish name derived from Agnes, symbolizing faith and spirituality.
- **Chapter:** 6

111. Ingrid 38
- **Meaning:** "beautiful" or "beloved"
- **Description:** Of Norse origin, Ingrid conveys strength and sophistication and is often linked to classic European elegance.
- **Chapter:** 2

112. Irene **20**
- **Meaning:** "peace"
- **Description:** A name of Greek origin tied to the goddess of peace, symbolizing harmony and serenity.
- **Chapter:** 2

113. Iris **76**
- **Meaning:** "rainbow"
- **Description:** A Greek name tied to the delicate flower and the goddess of the rainbow, symbolizing individuality and hope.
- **Chapter:** 4

114. Isabella **39**
- **Meaning:** "devoted to God"
- **Description:** A Hebrew and Italian name blending spirituality and beauty.
- **Chapter:** 2

115. Isla **76**
- **Meaning:** "island"
- **Description:** Of Scottish origin, Isla reflects serenity and natural beauty, evoking images of tranquil landscapes.
- **Chapter:** 4

116. Ivy **55**
- **Meaning:** "fidelity" or "friendship"
- **Description:** An English name symbolizing growth and loyalty, inspired by nature.

- **Chapter:** 3

117. Jade 76
- **Meaning:** "precious stone"
- **Description:** A British name representing beauty, wisdom, and prosperity, tied to the healing properties of the jade gemstone.
- **Chapter:** 4

118. Jane 33
- **Meaning:** "God is gracious"
- **Description:** A strong and elegant name tied to literary and historical figures like Jane Austen.
- **Chapter:** 2

119. Jasmine 39
- **Meaning:** "gift from God" or "jasmine flower"
- **Description:** Of Persian origin, Jasmine reflects beauty and grace, inspired by the fragrant and delicate flower.
- **Chapter:** 2

120. Jessica 21
- **Meaning:** "God beholds"
- **Description:** A name of Hebrew origin, popularized by Shakespeare in *The Merchant of Venice,* representing beauty and vision.
- **Chapter:** 2

121. Jillian 21

- **Meaning:** "youthful"
- **Description:** An English variation of Gillian, it combines classic charm with a playful modern twist.
- **Chapter:** 2

122. Joan 124
- **Meaning:** "God is gracious"
- **Description:** A Hebrew name tied to historical figures like Joan of Arc, representing resilience, courage, and divine grace.
- **Chapter:** 6

123. Jocelyn 131
- **Meaning:** "member of the Gauts tribe"
- **Description:** Of Old German origin, Jocelyn is a graceful name that became popular in medieval England and retains its elegance.
- **Chapter:** 6

124. Julia..34
- **Meaning:** "youthful" or "Jove's child"
- **Description:** A sophisticated and romantic name connected to literature and Roman mythology.
- **Chapter:** 2

125. Juliette 28
- **Meaning:** "youthful" or "soft-haired"

- **Description:** A French variation of Juliet, it evokes romance and refinement, tied to Shakespeare's *Romeo and Juliet*.
- **Chapter:** 2

126. Juniper 77
- **Meaning:** "evergreen"
- **Description:** A Latin name exuding vitality and growth, inspired by the aromatic tree.
- **Chapter:** 4

127. Juno 88
- **Meaning:** "queen of the gods"
- **Description:** A Latin name celebrating strength, loyalty, and protection, tied to Roman mythology.
- **Chapter:** 4

128. Katura 69
- **Meaning:** "crowned one"
- **Description:** A rare Hebrew name representing honor and grace, Katura carries a regal and ethereal quality.
- **Chapter:** 3

129. Kimberly 34
- **Meaning:** "from the meadow of the royal fortress"
- **Description:** An English name that became popular in the 20th century, symbolizing strength and charm.
- **Chapter:** 2

130. Kyoto **149**
- **Meaning:** "capital"
- **Description:** A Japanese name honoring the historical capital of Japan, symbolizing cultural and historical significance.
- **Chapter:** 7

131. Laura **21**
- **Meaning:** "bay laurel"
- **Description:** Of Latin origin, Laura signifies victory and honor, associated with the poetic muse and classic beauty.
- **Chapter:** 2

132. Layla **132**
- **Meaning:** "night"
- **Description:** Of Arabic origin, Layla is associated with beauty and mystery, popular in Middle Eastern and literary contexts.
- **Chapter:** 6

133. Leah **118**
- **Meaning:** "weary" or "delicate"
- **Description:** A Hebrew name tied to a matriarch in the Bible, symbolizing strength, endurance, and family loyalty.
- **Chapter:** 6

134. Leilani **77**
- **Meaning:** "heavenly garland of flowers"

- **Description:** Of Hawaiian origin, Leilani embodies grace and warmth, celebrating connection to nature and spiritual beauty.
- **Chapter:** 4

135. Lila 132
- **Meaning:** "night" or "divine play"
- **Description:** A multicultural name representing mystery, beauty, and creativity.
- **Chapter:** 6

136. Lillian 34
- **Meaning:** "lily"
- **Description:** Derived from the flower, this name signifies purity and elegance, making it a perennial favorite.
- **Chapter:** 2

137. Lily..77
- **Meaning:** "pure" or "lily flower"
- **Description:** A Latin name symbolizing innocence, grace, and renewal.
- **Chapter:** 4

138. Lourdes 140
- **Meaning:** "craggy slope"
- **Description:** A French name associated with the Marian apparition and pilgrimage site, symbolizing faith and healing.
- **Chapter:** 7

139. Lucia..28

- **Meaning:** "light"
- **Description:** Of Latin origin, Lucia is a radiant name associated with Saint Lucia, symbolizing brightness and clarity.
- **Chapter:** 2

140. Lucy 21
- **Meaning:** "light" or "light bringer"
- **Description:** A warm and timeless name symbolizing radiance and joy.
- **Chapter:** 2

141. Luna 88
- **Meaning:** "moon"
- **Description:** A Latin name embodying independence, radiance, and celestial beauty.
- **Chapter:** 4

142. Lyra 88
- **Meaning:** "lyre" or "lyre player"
- **Description:** A Greek name tied to music, creativity, and celestial beauty through the constellation Lyra.
- **Chapter:** 4

143. Madeline 43
- **Meaning:** "tower" or "from Magdala"
- **Description:** A Hebrew name symbolizing strength and steadfastness.
- **Chapter:** 2

144. Maeve 88

- **Meaning:** "intoxicating" or "she who rules"
- **Description:** An Irish name inspired by mythology, symbolizing beauty, power, and determination.
- **Chapter:** 4

145. Magnolia..77
- **Meaning:** "magnolia tree"
- **Description:** A French name symbolizing resilience, elegance, and natural grace.
- **Chapter:** 4

146. Maisie 50
- **Meaning:** "pearl"
- **Description:** A Scottish diminutive of Margaret, Maisie is sweet and endearing, with a vintage charm perfect for a spirited individual.
- **Chapter:** 3

147. Malia 124
- **Meaning:** "calm" or "peaceful"
- **Description:** Of Hawaiian origin, Malia is a serene and elegant name that carries a sense of harmony and natural beauty.
- **Chapter:** 6

148. Marbella 149
- **Meaning:** "fertile district"
- **Description:** A name tied to a Spanish coastal city, embodying Mediterranean charm and sophistication.

- **Chapter:** 7

149. Margaret 44
- **Meaning:** "pearl"
- **Description:** A Greek name representing purity and timeless elegance.
- **Chapter:** 2

150. Maria 39
- **Meaning:** "beloved" or "wished-for child"
- **Description:** A Latin name honoring faith, devotion, and universal grace.
- **Chapter:** 2

151. Marietta 149
- **Meaning:** "little Mary"
- **Description:** A diminutive of Mary, Marietta is of Italian origin, reflecting grace, devotion, and timeless charm.
- **Chapter:** 7

152. Maris 83
- **Meaning:** "of the sea"
- **Description:** A Latin name inspired by the beauty and mystery of the ocean, evoking calm and serenity.
- **Chapter:** 4

153. Marisol 62
- **Meaning:** "sea and sun"
- **Description:** A Spanish name evoking warmth, nature, and lyrical beauty.

- **Chapter:** 3

154. Martha 35
- **Meaning:** "lady" or "mistress"
- **Description:** Of Aramaic origin, Martha is a classic biblical name, symbolizing diligence and hospitality.
- **Chapter:** 2

155. Meadow 77
- **Meaning:** "open field"
- **Description:** A pastoral name evoking peace and natural beauty, inspired by serene landscapes.
- **Chapter:** 4

156. Melanie 21
- **Meaning:** "black" or "dark"
- **Description:** A Greek-origin name representing depth and mystery, popularized through Saint Melanie's legacy.
- **Chapter:** 2

157. Melissa 22
- **Meaning:** "bee"
- **Description:** Of Greek origin, Melissa ties to mythology, symbolizing nurturing qualities, productivity, and warmth.
- **Chapter:** 2

158. Meredith 44
- **Meaning:** "great ruler" or "sea lord"

- **Description:** A name of Welsh origin that balances strength and elegance, suitable for both modern and traditional tastes.
- **Chapter:** 2

159. Mia..78
- **Meaning:** "moon," "beloved," or "mine"
- **Description:** A name with Australian, Latin, and Scandinavian origins, symbolizing connection, affection, and the ocean's vast beauty.
- **Chapter:** 4

160. Michelle 22
- **Meaning:** "who is like God?"
- **Description:** A French feminine form of Michael, Michelle blends spiritual depth with a modern and graceful charm.
- **Chapter:** 2

161. Mira...56
- **Meaning:** "admirable" or "peace"
- **Description:** A multicultural name celebrating beauty, wisdom, and independence.
- **Chapter:** 3

162. Mireille 50
- **Meaning:** "to admire"
- **Description:** A French name embodying grace and charm.
- **Chapter:** 3

163. Miriam **125**
- **Meaning:** "wished-for child" or "sea of bitterness"
- **Description:** A Hebrew name tied to Moses's sister, representing courage and devotion.
- **Chapter:** 6

164. Molly..**35**
- **Meaning:** "bitter"
- **Description:** A diminutive of Mary, Molly is an endearing and approachable name with a lively, timeless charm.
- **Chapter:** 2

165. Monroe **149**
- **Meaning:** "mouth of the river"
- **Description:** A vintage name with Scottish roots, Monroe combines elegance with strength, ideal for a modern yet classic touch.
- **Chapter:** 7

166. Myra..**69**
- **Meaning:** "wonderful" or "admirable"
- **Description:** Of Greek origin, Myra represents qualities of excellence and beauty, offering a classic yet unique touch.
- **Chapter:** 3

167. Naomi..**40**
- **Meaning:** "pleasantness"

- **Description:** Of Hebrew origin, Naomi is a timeless biblical name symbolizing grace and kindness.
- **Chapter:** 2

168. Nara 140
- **Meaning:** "happy" or "nearest"
- **Description:** Of Japanese and Celtic origin, Nara symbolizes joy, closeness, and harmony, with ties to nature and ancient history.
- **Chapter:** 7

169. Nia 56
- **Meaning:** "purpose" or "brightness"
- **Description:** A Swahili and Welsh name symbolizing clarity, intention, and radiance.
- **Chapter:** 3

170. Nicole 22
- **Meaning:** "victory of the people"
- **Description:** Of Greek origin, Nicole is a refined name associated with grace and strength, often shortened to Nikki.
- **Chapter:** 2

171. Nina 62
- **Meaning:** "little girl" or "fire"
- **Description:** A versatile name with roots in Spanish, Native American, and Slavic traditions.
- **Chapter:** 3

172. Noemi..70
- **Meaning:** "pleasantness"
- **Description:** A Spanish and Italian form of Naomi, Noemi symbolizes grace and joy and is rooted in biblical tradition.
- **Chapter:** 3

173. Odessa...141
- **Meaning:** "long journey"
- **Description:** Rooted in Greek origins, Odessa is tied to the historic Ukrainian city, symbolizing resilience and cultural richness.
- **Chapter:** 7

174. Olivia 22
- **Meaning:** "olive tree"
- **Description:** A Latin name tied to peace and friendship, popularized by Shakespeare.
- **Chapter:** 2

175. Paloma..63
- **Meaning:** "dove"
- **Description:** A Spanish name symbolizing peace and purity, Paloma brings a serene and poetic appeal.
- **Chapter:** 3

176. Paris..141
- **Meaning:** "defender"
- **Description:** Linked to Greek mythology and the iconic French capital, Paris symbolizes

elegance, romance, and timeless sophistication.
- **Chapter:** 7

177. Penelope 44
- **Meaning:** "weaver" or "duck"
- **Description:** A Greek name symbolizing creativity and faithfulness, inspired by mythology.
- **Chapter:** 2

178. Petra 150
- **Meaning:** "rock"
- **Description:** Rooted in Greek origins, Petra evokes strength and resilience, tied to the stunning archaeological city in Jordan.
- **Chapter:** 7

179. Poppy...78
- **Meaning:** "peace" or "remembrance"
- **Description:** A Latin name associated with the vibrant and cheerful flower, symbolizing charm and depth.
- **Chapter:** 4

180. Priya 133
- **Meaning:** "beloved"
- **Description:** A Sanskrit name from India, symbolizing affection and cherished bonds.
- **Chapter:** 6

181. Rania 125

- **Meaning:** "queen" or "gazing"
- **Description:** Of Arabic origin, Rania signifies majesty and contemplation, often chosen for its regal and graceful tone.
- **Chapter:** 6

182. Raven 78
- **Meaning:** "large black bird"
- **Description:** A British name evoking mystery, intelligence, and individuality.
- **Chapter:** 4

183. Rebecca 29
- **Meaning:** "to tie" or "bind"
- **Description:** A Hebrew name with biblical significance, Rebecca represents beauty, faithfulness, and strength.
- **Chapter:** 2

184. Regina 40
- **Meaning:** "queen"
- **Description:** Of Latin origin, Regina signifies royalty and dignity, tied to strength and leadership.
- **Chapter:** 2

185. Renata 133
- **Meaning:** "reborn"
- **Description:** A Latin name symbolizing renewal and transformation, popular in various European cultures.
- **Chapter:** 6

186. Riona 70
- **Meaning:** "queenly" or "royal"
- **Description:** Of Irish origin, Riona represents nobility and strength, offering a regal and poetic charm.
- **Chapter:** 3

187. Rose 36
- **Meaning:** "flower"
- **Description:** A Latin name symbolizing beauty, love, and romance.
- **Chapter:** 2

188. Ruby 36
- **Meaning:** "red gemstone"
- **Description:** A vibrant name derived from the precious stone, symbolizing passion and vitality.
- **Chapter:** 2

189. Ruth 120
- **Meaning:** "friend"
- **Description:** A Hebrew name honoring the biblical heroine known for her loyalty and kindness.
- **Chapter:** 6

190. Saanvi 133
- **Meaning:** "goddess Lakshmi" or "summit"
- **Description:** An Indian name celebrating spiritual connection and ambition.

- **Chapter:** 6

191. Sahara **150**
- **Meaning:** "desert"
- **Description:** An Arabic-origin name celebrating the vast beauty of the Sahara Desert, evoking mystery and splendor.
- **Chapter:** 7

192. Sarah **40**
- **Meaning:** "princess"
- **Description:** A Hebrew name embodying nobility, grace, and strength.
- **Chapter:** 2

193. Saskia **63**
- **Meaning:** "protector of mankind"
- **Description:** A Dutch and German name associated with bravery and cultural richness.
- **Chapter:** 3

194. Savannah **142**
- **Meaning:** "from the open plain"
- **Description:** A Spanish and Native American name tied to Georgia's historic city, symbolizing exploration and natural beauty.
- **Chapter:** 7

195. Scarlett **134**
- **Meaning:** "red"

- **Description:** A French-origin name symbolizing passion, courage, and history, popularized by Scarlett O'Hara in *Gone with the Wind*.
- **Chapter:** 6

196. Selene..89
- **Meaning:** "the moon"
- **Description:** A Greek name tied to the moon goddess, symbolizing tranquility and ethereal beauty.
- **Chapter:** 4

197. Seraphim 120
- **Meaning:** "the burning one"
- **Description:** A Hebrew name referring to the highest-ranking angels, symbolizing divine strength and love.
- **Chapter:** 6

198. Serenity 120
- **Meaning:** "peaceful" or "calm"
- **Description:** A French virtue name embodying tranquility, grace, and inner strength.
- **Chapter:** 6

199. Sienna...142
- **Meaning:** "reddish-brown"
- **Description:** Inspired by the Italian city of Siena, this name reflects warmth, elegance, and artistic flair.

- **Chapter:** 3

200. Silvia 40
- **Meaning:** "forest"
- **Description:** Of Latin origin, Silvia connects to nature and serenity, symbolizing strength and tranquility.
- **Chapter:** 2

201. Simone 70
- **Meaning:** "one who hears"
- **Description:** Of French and Hebrew origins, Simone is a sophisticated and timeless name often associated with elegance and wisdom.
- **Chapter:** 3

202. Sol 79
- **Meaning:** "sun"
- **Description:** Of Spanish and Latin origin, Sol exudes warmth and radiance, symbolizing vitality and light.
- **Chapter:** 4

203. Sophia 29
- **Meaning:** "wisdom"
- **Description:** A name of beauty and intelligence, rooted in Greek philosophy and European royalty.
- **Chapter:** 2

204. Soraya 63
- **Meaning:** "Pleiades constellation"

- **Description:** Of Persian origin, Soraya embodies celestial beauty and mystique, offering a name full of grace and wonder.
- **Chapter:** 3

205. Stephanie 126
- **Meaning:** "crown" or "garland"
- **Description:** Of Greek origin, Stephanie is a classic and elegant name representing honor and victory.
- **Chapter:** 6

206. Summer 79
- **Meaning:** "season of warmth and sunshine"
- **Description:** Of Old English origin, Summer signifies vitality and joy, bringing to mind carefree days and vibrant energy.
- **Chapter:** 4

207. Susanna 29
- **Meaning:** "lily"
- **Description:** A biblical name of Hebrew origin symbolizing purity and grace, often shortened to Susie or Anna.
- **Chapter:** 2

208. Sydney 146
- **Meaning:** "Saint Denis" or "dweller by the well-watered land"
- **Description:** A French and British-origin name tied to the Australian city, symbolizing creativity and innovation.

- **Chapter:** 7

209. Sylvan 79
- **Meaning:** "of the forest"
- **Description:** A Latin name inspired by the Roman god of forests, symbolizing harmony and mystery.
- **Chapter:** 4

210. Tabitha 121
- **Meaning:** "gazelle"
- **Description:** A biblical name symbolizing grace and beauty, tied to a compassionate figure in the New Testament.
- **Chapter:** 6

211. Talia 121
- **Meaning:** "dew from heaven" or "blooming"
- **Description:** Of Hebrew and Greek origin, Talia reflects serenity and divine blessings, offering a soft and melodic sound.
- **Chapter:** 6

212. Theresa 126
- **Meaning:** "summer" or "to harvest"
- **Description:** A Greek name reflecting life cycles, associated with Saint Teresa and Mother Teresa.
- **Chapter:** 6

213. Thora 89
- **Meaning:** "thunder"

- **Description:** A Scandinavian name honoring strength and protection, tied to Norse mythology.
- **Chapter:** 4

214. Tove 64
- **Meaning:** "beautiful" or "dove"
- **Description:** A Scandinavian name with Nordic charm, Tove combines simplicity with elegance, symbolizing peace and beauty.
- **Chapter:** 3

215. Valencia 142
- **Meaning:** "strength"
- **Description:** A name celebrating the Spanish coastal city, embodying energy, vibrancy, and a zest for life.
- **Chapter:** 7

216. Valentina 134
- **Meaning:** "strong" or "healthy"
- **Description:** A Latin name associated with love, resilience, and Saint Valentine's Day.
- **Chapter:** 6

217. Vanessa 41
- **Meaning:** "butterfly"
- **Description:** A literary name coined by Jonathan Swift, Vanessa symbolizes transformation, beauty, and creativity.
- **Chapter:** 2

218. Verona..**142**
- **Meaning:** "truth"
- **Description:** Verona reflects the charm of Shakespeare's romantic setting in *Romeo and Juliet*, perfect for lovers of literature and history.
- **Chapter:** 7

219. Veronica..**30**
- **Meaning:** "true image"
- **Description:** Of Latin and Greek origin, Veronica is a name with religious and artistic associations, symbolizing faith and virtue.
- **Chapter:** 2

220. Vesta..**89**
- **Meaning:** "hearth"
- **Description:** A Latin name symbolizing warmth, family, and protection, tied to Roman mythology.
- **Chapter:** 4

221. Victoria..**23**
- **Meaning:** "victory"
- **Description:** A name of strength and triumph that is tied to Queen Victoria and Roman mythology.
- **Chapter:** 2

222. Vienna..**142**

- **Meaning:** "from the city of Vienna"
- **Description:** A name inspired by Austria's capital, known for its music, art, and cultural vibrance.
- **Chapter:** 7

223. Violet 79
- **Meaning:** "purple" or "violet flower"
- **Description:** A Latin name reflecting beauty, grace, and romantic charm.
- **Chapter:** 4

224. Willow 80
- **Meaning**: "willow tree"
- **Description**: Of British origin, Willow symbolizes adaptability and quiet strength, reflecting the natural elegance of the tree's flowing branches.
- **Chapter:** 4

225. Winter 83
- **Meaning:** "time of water"
- **Description:** A British and German name evoking the beauty and transformation of the season.
- **Chapter:** 4

226. Yara 134
- **Meaning:** "small butterfly" or "water lady"
- **Description:** A cross-cultural name symbolizing strength, beauty, and companionship.

- **Chapter:** 6

227. Yasmin 64
- **Meaning:** "jasmine flower"
- **Description:** Of Persian origin, Yasmin evokes floral beauty and a gentle, fragrant charm, symbolizing grace and purity.
- **Chapter:** 3

228. Zaira 71
- **Meaning:** "brightness" or "blooming flower"
- **Description:** An Arabic name symbolizing natural beauty and radiance.
- **Chapter:** 3

229. Zara 64
- **Meaning:** "princess" or "radiance"
- **Description:** Of Arabic and Hebrew origins, Zara is a chic and vibrant name signifying beauty and brightness.
- **Chapter:** 3

230. Zinnia 84
- **Meaning:** "bold flower"
- **Description:** A German name symbolizing endurance, affection, and vibrant spirit.
- **Chapter:** 4

231. Zoey 52
- **Meaning:** "life"

- **Description:** Of Greek origin, Zoey is a lively and modern name symbolizing vitality and energy, making it a joyful choice.
- **Chapter:** 3

232. Zola 134
- **Meaning:** "earth" or "calm"
- **Description:** Of African and Italian origins, Zola reflects a connection to nature and serenity.
- **Chapter:** 6

233. Zuri 58
- **Meaning:** "beautiful"
- **Description:** A Swahili name celebrating elegance and life's preciousness.
- **Chapter:** 3

Gender-Neutral Names

1. Addison 96
- **Meaning:** "son of Adam"
- **Description:** Of Old English origin, Addison has evolved into a stylish, modern name, symbolizing strength and individuality.
- **Chapter:** 5

2. Aeron 81
- **Meaning:** "berry" or "battle"

- **Description:** A Welsh name tied to nature and mythology, reflecting resilience and grace.
- **Chapter:** 4

3. Akira 128
- **Meaning:** "bright" or "intelligent"
- **Description:** A Japanese name reflecting brilliance and clarity and also linked to stability.
- **Chapter:** 6

4. Alaska 143
- **Meaning:** "great land"
- **Description:** This name celebrates the untamed beauty and adventurous spirit of the northernmost U.S. state.
- **Chapter:** 7

5. Alexis 101
- **Meaning:** "helper" or "defender"
- **Description:** Of Greek origin, Alexis is a strong and versatile name, symbolizing protection and compassion.
- **Chapter:** 5

6. Anden 144
- **Meaning:** "spirit" or "breath"
- **Description:** Tied to the Andes Mountains, this Scandinavian name evokes grandeur and natural beauty.
- **Chapter:** 7

7. Archer..105
- **Meaning:** "bowman"
- **Description:** Of English origin, Archer conveys skill and precision, symbolizing strength and focus. It's a modern name with historical ties to craftsmanship and adventure.
- **Chapter:** 5

8. Arden 96
- **Meaning:** "valley of the eagle"
- **Description:** Of Celtic origin, Arden reflects nature and independence, evoking strength and grace.
- **Chapter:** 5

9. Ari 59
- **Meaning:** "lion" or "eagle"
- **Description:** A Hebrew and Norse name symbolizing strength, freedom, and resilience.
- **Chapter:** 3

10. Ariel...115
- **Meaning**: "lion of God"
- **Description**: Of Hebrew origin, Ariel is a versatile name tied to strength and divinity, often linked to nature and spiritual protection.
- **Chapter:** 6

11. Arlo **105**
- **Meaning:** "fortified hill" or "barberry tree"
- **Description:** Of Old English and Spanish origins, Arlo conveys a rustic charm and free-spirited vibe. Its simplicity and soft sound make it a modern favorite.
- **Chapter:** 5

12. Aspen **74**
- **Meaning:** "aspen tree"
- **Description:** A gender-neutral name reflecting resilience and transformation, inspired by the heart-shaped leaves of the aspen tree.
- **Chapter:** 4

13. Avery **92**
- **Meaning:** "elf counsel" or "ruler of elves"
- **Description:** A British-origin name with a magical connotation, balancing whimsy and modern appeal.
- **Chapter:** 5

14. Baylor **97**
- **Meaning:** "deliverer of goods"
- **Description:** Of Old English origin, Baylor reflects practicality and resourcefulness, offering a strong yet approachable modern feel.
- **Chapter:** 5

15. Blair **148**

- **Meaning:** "field"
- **Description:** A sleek Scottish name tied to serene landscapes, symbolizing peace and elegance.
- **Chapter:** 7

16. Blake...106
- **Meaning:** "dark," "black," or "pale"
- **Description:** A British-origin name symbolizing balance and duality, with modern artistic connections.
- **Chapter:** 5

17. Blaze..81
- **Meaning:** "fire" or "flame"
- **Description:** A Latin name embodying passion, energy, and individuality.
- **Chapter:** 4

18. Braxton 101
- **Meaning:** "brock's town"
- **Description:** Derived from Old English, Braxton reflects boldness and individuality, offering a modern, edgy feel.
- **Chapter:** 5

19. Briar 75
- **Meaning:** "thorny bush of wild roses"
- **Description:** A British name symbolizing strength and beauty.
- **Chapter:** 4

20. Brooklyn..................................**144**
- **Meaning:** "small stream"
- **Description:** A modern, artistic name tied to the New York City borough, celebrating individuality and creativity.
- **Chapter:** 7

21. Calais......................................**148**
- **Meaning:** "changing color"
- **Description:** A gender-neutral name tied to the French port city, symbolizing transformation and versatility.
- **Chapter:** 7

22. Callum....................................**106**
- **Meaning:** "dove"
- **Description:** Of Scottish origin, Callum symbolizes peace and serenity. Its soft yet steadfast nature makes it a timeless choice with a gentle appeal.
- **Chapter:** 5

23. Camden..................................**106**
- **Meaning:** "winding valley"
- **Description:** Of Scottish and Old English origin, Camden ties nature to charm, offering a fresh and contemporary sound with historical depth.
- **Chapter:** 5

24. Cameron................................**109**
- **Meaning:** "crooked nose"

- **Description:** A Scottish-origin name linked to leadership and resilience, widely embraced for its adaptability.
- **Chapter:** 5

25. Carson 144
- **Meaning:** "son of the marsh-dwellers"
- **Description:** A versatile and approachable name that blends historical roots with modern appeal.
- **Chapter:** 7

26. Carter..101
- **Meaning:** "transporter of goods by cart"
- **Description:** A British-origin name associated with hard work and creativity, blending tradition and modernity.
- **Chapter:** 5

27. Casey..92
- **Meaning:** "vigilant" or "watchful"
- **Description:** Of Irish origin, Casey symbolizes attentiveness and strength, with a timeless and adaptable quality that suits any gender.
- **Chapter:** 5

28. Cedar...75
- **Meaning:** "cedar tree"
- **Description:** A name of strength and longevity, inspired by the sacred and protective qualities of the cedar tree.

- **Chapter:** 4

29. Chase..106
- **Meaning:** "hunter"
- **Description:** Of French origin, Chase reflects energy and adventure and is often associated with determination and focus.
- **Chapter:** 5

30. Chelsea..139
- **Meaning:** "port of ships"
- **Description:** Of Old English origin, Chelsea represents connection to the sea, evoking elegance and sophistication.
- **Chapter:** 7

31. Cove..81
- **Meaning:** "small coastal inlet"
- **Description:** A British name reflecting serenity, adventure, and calm strength.
- **Chapter:** 4

32. Crew 102
- **Meaning:** "a group of people" or "chariot"
- **Description:** Of English and Latin origin, Crew reflects unity and collaboration. Its concise, modern sound has made it a stylish and contemporary choice.
- **Chapter:** 5

33. Cypress 75
- **Meaning:** "cypress tree"

- **Description:** A Greek name symbolizing endurance, grace, and protection.
- **Chapter:** 4

34. Dakota..145
- **Meaning:** "friend" or "ally"
- **Description:** A Native American name celebrating loyalty and bravery, with connections to the Great Plains.
- **Chapter:** 7

35. Dawsen..106
- **Meaning:** "son of David"
- **Description:** A modern variant of Dawson, this name has biblical ties and represents legacy and strength, with a contemporary twist.
- **Chapter:** 5

36. Devon..148
- **Meaning**: "from the valley"
- **Description**: Of English origin, Devon is a fresh and adaptable name tied to nature and adventure.
- **Chapter:** 7

37. Dylan..109
- **Meaning:** "great tide" or "son of the sea"
- **Description:** A Welsh name with deep connections to water, symbolizing adaptability and resilience.
- **Chapter:** 5

38. Easton 102
- **Meaning:** "east-facing place"
- **Description:** Of English origin, Easton reflects direction and opportunity, making it a modern name that carries aspirations and optimism.
- **Chapter:** 5

39. Eden 116
- **Meaning:** "delight" or "place of pleasure"
- **Description:** A biblical name referring to the Garden of Eden, representing purity and a divine sanctuary.
- **Chapter:** 6

40. Ellis 109
- **Meaning:** "kind" or "benevolent"
- **Description:** A name with Welsh, Greek, and Hebrew roots, symbolizing inclusivity and compassion.
- **Chapter:** 5

41. Ember 82
- **Meaning:** "spark" or "burning low"
- **Description:** A gender-neutral name evoking warmth and resilience, inspired by the glowing remains of a fire.
- **Chapter:** 4

42. Emerson 93
- **Meaning:** "son of Emery"

- **Description:** Of German origin, Emerson conveys industriousness and strength. Its versatility makes it a favorite for parents seeking a gender-neutral name.
- **Chapter:** 5

43. Emery 93
- **Meaning:** "industrious ruler"
- **Description:** Of German origin, Emery represents strength and leadership, blending tradition with modern charm.
- **Chapter:** 5

44. Everest 145
- **Meaning:** "dweller on the Eure River"
- **Description:** A bold name linked to the tallest mountain in the world, symbolizing strength and achievement.
- **Chapter:** 7

45. Fallon 97
- **Meaning:** "leader"
- **Description:** Of Irish origin, Fallon embodies strength and charisma. Its bold and energetic feel makes it a standout choice for modern parents.
- **Chapter:** 5

46. Finley 93
- **Meaning:** "fair-haired hero"

- **Description:** Of Irish origin, Finley combines traditional roots with modern versatility, offering a timeless appeal for any gender.
- **Chapter:** 5

47. Finn...97

- **Meaning:** "fair" or "blessed"
- **Description:** An Irish and Scandinavian name with mythological roots, symbolizing wisdom and leadership.
- **Chapter:** 5

48. Francis 43

- **Meaning:** "free man"
- **Description:** A Latin name reflecting humility, kindness, and strength.
- **Chapter:** 2

49. Gia 106

- **Meaning:** "God's gracious gift"
- **Description:** Of Italian origin, Gia offers elegance in simplicity, symbolizing gratitude and divine grace.
- **Chapter:** 5

50. Grant 109

- **Meaning**: "great"
- **Description**: Of Scottish origin, Grant signifies generosity and grandeur, embodying strength and dignity.
- **Chapter:** 5

51. Gray 97
- **Meaning:** "gray-haired" or "gray"
- **Description:** A modern, color-inspired name of Old English origin, Gray is sleek and understated, exuding sophistication and neutrality.
- **Chapter:** 5

52. Hallie 110
- **Meaning:** "dweller at the hall meadow"
- **Description:** Of Old English origin, Hallie is a bright and cheerful name that reflects nature and harmony.
- **Chapter:** 5

53. Harlow 93
- **Meaning:** "rocky hill"
- **Description:** Of Old English origin, Harlow offers a mix of natural beauty and strength, symbolizing resilience and elegance.
- **Chapter:** 5

54. Harmony 117
- **Meaning:** "unity" or "concord"
- **Description:** A virtue name symbolizing balance and peace, often chosen for its connection to music and togetherness.
- **Chapter:** 6

55. Harper 97
- **Meaning:** "harpist" or "minstrel"

- **Description:** A British-origin name celebrating creativity and harmony, with strong artistic associations.
- **Chapter:** 5

56. Havana 145
- **Meaning:** "of the Habana people"
- **Description:** A unique name tied to Cuba's capital, symbolizing cultural depth and historical legacy.
- **Chapter:** 7

57. Haven 139
- **Meaning:** "safe place"
- **Description:** An Old English name symbolizing comfort, security, and love.
- **Chapter:** 7

58. Hayden 98
- **Meaning:** "heather-covered hill"
- **Description:** Of Old English origin, Hayden symbolizes connection to nature and resilience, offering a contemporary sound.
- **Chapter:** 5

59. Hendrix 102
- **Meaning:** "son of Hendrick"
- **Description:** Of Dutch and German origin, Hendrix reflects creativity and individuality, famously tied to musical icon Jimi Hendrix.
- **Chapter:** 5

60. Hollis 110
- **Meaning:** "holly trees"
- **Description:** A British-origin name evoking natural beauty and resilience, with festive undertones.
- **Chapter:** 5

61. Hudson 102
- **Meaning:** "son of Hugh"
- **Description:** Of English origin, Hudson combines strength and heritage, often associated with the iconic Hudson River.
- **Chapter:** 5

62. Hunter 102
- **Meaning:** "one who hunts"
- **Description:** A British-origin name symbolizing independence, resourcefulness, and a connection to nature.
- **Chapter:** 5

63. Imani 130
- **Meaning:** "belief" or "faith"
- **Description:** A Swahili and Arabic name inspiring trust, optimism, and spiritual depth.
- **Chapter:** 6

64. Indigo 69
- **Meaning:** "deep blue dye"

- **Description:** Of Greek and English origin, Indigo evokes creativity and depth, symbolizing individuality and vibrancy.
- **Chapter:** 3

65. Jett 102
- **Meaning**: "black mineral"
- **Description**: Of English origin, Jett exudes sleek modernity and boldness, symbolizing energy and individuality.
- **Chapter:** 5

66. Jordan 93
- **Meaning:** "to flow down" or "descending"
- **Description:** A biblical name tied to the River Jordan, symbolizing strength and adaptability.
- **Chapter:** 5

67. Jovie 110
- **Meaning:** "joyful"
- **Description:** Of American origin, Jovie is cheerful and lively, bringing a modern twist to traditional names symbolizing happiness.
- **Chapter:** 5

68. Jubilee 118
- **Meaning:** "year of celebration"
- **Description:** A biblical name representing joy and freedom, derived from the Jewish tradition of the jubilee year.
- **Chapter:** 6

69. Jude 103
- **Meaning:** "praised"
- **Description:** Of Hebrew origin, Jude is a strong, concise name with biblical ties, embodying praise and steadfastness.
- **Chapter:** 5

70. Kai 107
- **Meaning:** "sea" (Hawaiian), "food" (Māori), and "victory" (Japanese)
- **Description:** A globally appealing name symbolizing harmony, nature, and nourishment.
- **Chapter:** 5

71. Keegan 110
- **Meaning:** "descendant of Aodhagán"
- **Description:** Of Irish origin, Keegan symbolizes fire and passion, offering a bold and charismatic modern feel.
- **Chapter:** 5

72. Kendall 93
- **Meaning:** "valley of the River Kent"
- **Description:** Of Old English origin, Kendall balances natural beauty with modern versatility, making it a sleek choice.
- **Chapter:** 5

73. Kieran 56
- **Meaning:** "little dark one"

- **Description:** Of Irish origin, Kieran combines tradition with versatility, reflecting strength and individuality.
- **Chapter:** 3

74. Kiran 98
- **Meaning:** "ray of light"
- **Description:** Of Sanskrit origin, Kiran is a luminous and uplifting name, tied to clarity and inspiration.
- **Chapter:** 5

75. Knox 103
- **Meaning:** "hill"
- **Description:** Of Scottish origin, Knox exudes strength and simplicity, offering a modern, rugged appeal tied to nature.
- **Chapter:** 5

76. Landon 103
- **Meaning:** "long hill"
- **Description:** Of Old English origin, Landon evokes stability and a connection to nature, symbolizing growth and resilience.
- **Chapter:** 5

77. Landry 98
- **Meaning:** "ruler"
- **Description:** Of French origin, Landry symbolizes leadership and resilience, offering a unique yet timeless choice.
- **Chapter:** 5

78. Leighton **98**
- **Meaning:** "meadow town"
- **Description:** Of Old English origin, Leighton combines natural charm with elegance, offering a sophisticated yet approachable feel.
- **Chapter:** 5

79. Lennon **103**
- **Meaning:** "lover"
- **Description:** Of Irish origin, Lennon is a modern name tied to creativity and music and is often associated with the legacy of John Lennon.
- **Chapter:** 5

80. Leslie **98**
- **Meaning:** "holly garden"
- **Description:** Of Scottish origin, Leslie ties nature with grace, offering a versatile and timeless name that suits any gender.
- **Chapter:** 5

81. Lin **107**
- **Meaning:** "forest" or "fine jade"
- **Description:** A Chinese-origin name celebrating nature, brightness, and serenity.
- **Chapter:** 5

82. Lincoln **107**
- **Meaning:** "lake colony"

- **Description:** Of Old English origin, Lincoln represents history and strength, famously tied to U.S. President Abraham Lincoln.
- **Chapter:** 5

83. Logan 98
- **Meaning:** "hollow"
- **Description:** A Scottish-origin name blending strength, independence, and modern appeal.
- **Chapter:** 5

84. London 140
- **Meaning:** "from the great river"
- **Description:** Celebrating England's bustling capital, London reflects sophistication, history, and modern vibrancy.
- **Chapter:** 7

85. Luca 99
- **Meaning:** "bringer of light"
- **Description:** Of Latin origin, Luca combines warmth and brightness, often associated with inspiration and kindness.
- **Chapter:** 5

86. Maddox 103
- **Meaning:** "son of Madoc"
- **Description:** Of Welsh origin, Maddox combines tradition with boldness, offering a modern edge with historical significance.
- **Chapter:** 5

87. Maren...99
- **Meaning:** "sea"
- **Description:** Of Latin origin, Maren reflects tranquility and nature, symbolizing beauty and depth.
- **Chapter:** 5

88. Max 107
- **Meaning:** "greatest"
- **Description:** Short for Maximilian, this Latin-derived name is bold, timeless, and packed with strength and significance.
- **Chapter:** 5

89. Memphis 140
- **Meaning:** "enduring beauty"
- **Description:** Named after the ancient Egyptian city and the lively Tennessee city, Memphis symbolizes history and rhythm.
- **Chapter:** 7

90. Mika..62
- **Meaning:** "who is like God?" or "beautiful fragrance"
- **Description:** With roots in Hebrew and Japanese, Mika is a short and sweet name reflecting versatility and beauty.
- **Chapter:** 3

91. Milan 149
- **Meaning:** "gracious" or "kind"

- **Description:** A Slavic name associated with the Italian city, Milan represents sophistication and creativity.
- **Chapter:** 7

92. Milo 103
- **Meaning:** "soldier" or "merciful"
- **Description:** Of Latin and Germanic origins, Milo combines strength and kindness, offering a name that feels both historic and modern.
- **Chapter:** 5

93. Montana 150
- **Meaning:** "mountain"
- **Description:** A Latin name symbolizing resilience and adventure, associated with the majestic landscapes of the U.S. state.
- **Chapter:** 7

94. Morgan 99
- **Meaning:** "circling sea"
- **Description:** A Welsh name tied to nature and Celtic mythology, symbolizing strength and adventure.
- **Chapter:** 5

95. Nash 110
- **Meaning:** "by the ash tree"
- **Description:** Of English origin, Nash combines nature with simplicity, offering a strong yet gentle modern choice.

- **Chapter:** 5

96. Nico 99
- **Meaning:** "victory of the people"
- **Description:** A sleek, Greek-derived name that conveys strength and adaptability.
- **Chapter:** 5

97. Noelle 107
- **Meaning:** "Christmas"
- **Description:** Of French origin, Noelle exudes festivity and warmth, symbolizing joy and celebration.
- **Chapter:** 5

98. Nova 104
- **Meaning:** "new"
- **Description:** A Latin-origin name with celestial associations, symbolizing innovation and brightness.
- **Chapter:** 5

99. Onyx 111
- **Meaning:** "black gemstone"
- **Description:** Of Greek origin, Onyx symbolizes strength, resilience, and mystery, making it a bold and distinctive choice.
- **Chapter:** 5

100. Ori 108

- **Meaning:** "my light" (Hebrew), "cherry blossom" (Japanese), and "destiny" (Yoruba)
- **Description:** A multicultural name symbolizing guidance, nature, and intuition.
- **Chapter:** 5

101. Oslo 150

- **Meaning:** "estuary" or "meadow of the gods"
- **Description:** A Scandinavian-inspired name tied to Norway's capital, offering cultural significance and charm.
- **Chapter:** 7

102. Paisley 111

- **Meaning:** "patterned fabric"
- **Description:** Of Scottish origin, Paisley symbolizes creativity and charm, evoking artistic expression and individuality.
- **Chapter:** 5

103. Parker 99

- **Meaning:** "park keeper"
- **Description:** A British-origin name tied to nature, symbolizing freedom and playfulness.
- **Chapter:** 5

104. Paxton 104

- **Meaning:** "peace town"

- **Description:** Of Latin origin, Paxton represents harmony and community, offering a modern yet grounded feel.
- **Chapter:** 5

105. Peyton 100
- **Meaning:** "fighter's estate"
- **Description:** Of Old English origin, Peyton combines strength and sophistication, offering versatility and modern appeal.
- **Chapter:** 5

106. Phoenix 83
- **Meaning:** "rebirth"
- **Description:** A Greek name representing transformation, strength, and resilience, inspired by the legendary bird.
- **Chapter:** 4

107. Piper 56
- **Meaning:** "flute player"
- **Description:** Of English origin, Piper is a lively, modern name inspired by musical traditions and creativity.
- **Chapter:** 3

108. Presley 100
- **Meaning:** "priest's meadow"
- **Description:** Of English origin, Presley ties nature to creativity and is famously linked to music legend Elvis Presley.

- **Chapter:** 5

109. Quinley 51
- **Meaning:** "son of the hound of Leinster"
- **Description:** An Irish-inspired unisex name, Quinley combines tradition with a playful modern twist, symbolizing loyalty and joy.
- **Chapter:** 3

110. Quinn 104
- **Meaning:** "chief," "counsel," or "wisdom"
- **Description:** A Gaelic name celebrating leadership and intelligence with a sleek, modern sound.
- **Chapter:** 5

111. Raelyn 94
- **Meaning:** "beam of light" or "advisor"
- **Description:** A modern combination name of Hebrew and English origins, Raelyn blends warmth with wisdom, making it a heartfelt choice.
- **Chapter:** 5

112. Rain 83
- **Meaning:** "abundance from above"
- **Description:** A gentle name representing renewal, growth, and nurturing qualities.
- **Chapter:** 4

113. Reese 104

- **Meaning:** "enthusiasm" or "fire"
- **Description:** A Welsh name brimming with passion and charisma.
- **Chapter:** 5

114. Remington..111
- **Meaning:** "settlement by the riverbank"
- **Description:** Of English origin, Remington reflects adaptability and strength, often associated with sophistication and elegance.
- **Chapter:** 5

115. Remy 141
- **Meaning:** "from Rheims"
- **Description:** A French name symbolizing sophistication and cultural depth.
- **Chapter:** 7

116. Rhett 111
- **Meaning:** "advisor"
- **Description:** Of Dutch origin, Rhett reflects wisdom and confidence, offering a suave, modern feel with historical roots.
- **Chapter:** 5

117. Rhodes 141
- **Meaning:** "where roses grow"
- **Description:** Of Greek origin, Rhodes is tied to the beautiful Aegean island, symbolizing beauty, strength, and cultural legacy.

- **Chapter:** 7

118. Riley..94
- **Meaning:** "courageous" or "rye clearing"
- **Description:** Of Irish origin, Riley is a versatile name symbolizing resilience and bravery.
- **Chapter:** 5

119. Rio...146
- **Meaning:** "river"
- **Description:** A Spanish name reflecting flowing energy and the vibrant Brazilian city, Rio de Janeiro.
- **Chapter:** 7

120. Rory 100
- **Meaning:** "red king"
- **Description:** Of Irish and Scottish origin, Rory conveys leadership and vitality, offering a strong yet playful appeal.
- **Chapter:** 5

121. Rowan..94
- **Meaning:** "little redhead" or "rowan tree"
- **Description:** An Irish and Scottish name symbolizing protection, strength, and enchantment.
- **Chapter:** 5

122. Ryan...100
- **Meaning:** "little king"

- **Description:** Of Irish origin, Ryan reflects strength and leadership, embodying a blend of tradition and modern versatility.
- **Chapter:** 5

123. Sage 78
- **Meaning:** "wise" or "prophet"
- **Description:** A Latin name celebrating intellect, insight, and clarity.
- **Chapter:** 4

124. Salem 150
- **Meaning:** "peace"
- **Description:** Rooted in Hebrew origins, Salem symbolizes tranquility and history, tied to the Massachusetts city and its colonial legacy.
- **Chapter:** 7

125. Sasha 111
- **Meaning:** "defender of mankind"
- **Description:** Of Russian and Greek origin, Sasha is a charming, gender-neutral name with a modern and global flair.
- **Chapter:** 5

126. Sawyer 94
- **Meaning:** "woodcutter"
- **Description:** Of English origin, Sawyer represents resilience and craftsmanship, tied to literary and adventurous associations.

- **Chapter:** 5

127. Saylor...94
- **Meaning:** "dancer" or "acrobat"
- **Description:** Of German origin, Saylor represents adventure and creativity, making it a modern, free-spirited choice.
- **Chapter:** 5

128. Scout...95
- **Meaning:** "one who gathers information"
- **Description:** Of French origin, Scout is playful and adventurous, symbolizing curiosity and exploration.
- **Chapter:** 5

129. Selah 120
- **Meaning:** "pause and reflect"
- **Description:** A Hebrew name from the Psalms, signifying contemplation and spiritual depth.
- **Chapter:** 6

130. Shiloh..120
- **Meaning:** "tranquil" or "His gift"
- **Description:** A Hebrew name tied to a place of peace and divine assembly, symbolizing serenity and spiritual abundance.
- **Chapter:** 6

131. Silas..111

- **Meaning:** "forest" or "wood"
- **Description:** Of Latin origin, Silas embodies nature and tranquility, offering a timeless and grounded appeal.
- **Chapter:** 5

132. Sky..79
- **Meaning:** "atmosphere seen from Earth"
- **Description:** A Scandinavian name reflecting freedom, vastness, and inspiration.
- **Chapter:** 4

133. Skyler..95
- **Meaning:** "scholar"
- **Description:** Of Dutch origin, Skyler combines intellect and modern charm, appealing as a creative name.
- **Chapter:** 5

134. Sloan...112
- **Meaning:** "raider" or "warrior"
- **Description:** An Irish-origin name embodying courage, resilience, and heritage.
- **Chapter:** 5

135. Suki..134
- **Meaning:** "beloved"
- **Description:** A Japanese name emphasizing love and affection, often

chosen for its gentle and endearing qualities.
- **Chapter:** 6

136. Sutton 95
- **Meaning:** "southern settlement"
- **Description:** Of Old English origin, Sutton reflects heritage and direction, offering a sophisticated yet modern charm.
- **Chapter:** 5

137. Tahiti 151
- **Meaning:** "little king Hiro"
- **Description:** A Polynesian name tied to the breathtaking island, embodying natural beauty and mythology.
- **Chapter:** 7

138. Tahoe..146
- **Meaning:** "edge of the lake"
- **Description:** A serene and nature-inspired name tied to the stunning Lake Tahoe, symbolizing tranquility and adventure.
- **Chapter:** 7

139. Tanner 108
- **Meaning:** "leather worker"
- **Description:** Of Old English origin, Tanner reflects craftsmanship and resilience, offering a rugged yet modern feel.
- **Chapter:** 5

140. Tate..108
- **Meaning:** "cheerful"
- **Description:** A British-origin name symbolizing positivity and approachability, with a timeless charm.
- **Chapter:** 5

141. Tatum 100
- **Meaning:** "Tate's homestead"
- **Description:** Of Old English origin, Tatum symbolizes tradition and warmth, with a light and contemporary sound.
- **Chapter:** 5

142. Taylor 95
- **Meaning:** "tailor" or "to cut"
- **Description:** A French-origin name symbolizing precision and artistry.
- **Chapter:** 5

143. Teagan 95
- **Meaning:** "little poet"
- **Description:** Of Irish origin, Teagan reflects creativity and wisdom, offering a name that is lyrical and meaningful.
- **Chapter:** 5

144. Tyler 36
- **Meaning:** "tile maker"

- **Description**: Of Old English origin, Tyler is a modern yet classic name, representing craftsmanship and resourcefulness.
- **Chapter**: 2

145. Vesper 70
- **Meaning**: "evening star" or "evening prayer"
- **Description**: A Latin name symbolizing tranquility, peace, and celestial beauty.
- **Chapter**: 3

146. Waverly 52
- **Meaning**: "meadow of quivering aspens"
- **Description**: Of English origin, Waverly evokes imagery of natural beauty and tranquility, offering a unique yet gentle choice.
- **Chapter**: 3

147. Wren 95
- **Meaning**: "small bird"
- **Description**: Of English origin, Wren symbolizes freedom and nature, making it a simple yet elegant choice for modern parents.
- **Chapter**: 5

148. Zephyr 83
- **Meaning**: "west wind"

- **Description:** A Greek name symbolizing growth, renewal, and the mild breezes of spring.
- **Chapter:** 4

149. Zion 104
- **Meaning:** "highest point"
- **Description:** A Hebrew name with deep spiritual roots, symbolizing hope, resilience, and achievement.
- **Chapter:** 5

References

Barrett, J. (2010, March 13). *Baby names: Does popularity affect choice?* Newsweek. https://www.newsweek.com/baby-names-does-popularity-affect-choice-89937

CBS Newsroom. (2016, May 11). *Yes, there's now science behind naming your baby.* Columbia Business School. https://business.columbia.edu/press-releases/cbs-press-releases/yes-theres-now-science-behind-naming-your-baby

McAndrew, F. T. (2020, October 5). Why the choice of your child's name matters so much. *Psychology Today.* https://www.psychologytoday.com/za/blog/out-of-the-ooze/202010/why-the-choice-of-your-childs-name-matters-so-much

Moss, J. (2024, December 18). *Meaning of the name Mallory.* BabyNames.com. https://babynames.com/name/mallory

Obie Editorial Team. *(n.d.) How to choose a baby name to fit your last name.* babyMed. https://babymed.com/baby-names/choosing-a-baby-name-to-fit-your-last-name

Sharmaa, C. (2023, August 28). 15 unique Indian baby names starting with 'A' and the profound insights of numerologist Chandresh Sharmaa.

Vaastu & Numero Expert Chandresh Sharmaa. https://vaastu-numerology.com/15-unique-indian-baby-names-starting-with-a-and-the-profound-insights-of-numerologist-chandresh-sharmaa/

Thompson, S. (2024, September 27). *100+ Japanese names that mean "flower" and their meanings.* Paige Simple. https://www.paigesimple.org/japanese-names-that-mean-flower/

Vincentelli, E. (2007, November 4). *You are what your name says you are.* The New York Times. https://www.nytimes.com/2007/11/04/weekinreview/04vincentelli.html

Zhang, S. (2023, March 23). *The rise of gender-neutral names isn't what it seems.* The Atlantic. https://www.theatlantic.com/science/archive/2023/03/gender-neutral-baby-names-popularity/673464/

Made in the USA
Coppell, TX
29 April 2025